Learning Instructions and Exercises of
Human Regional Anatomy

主　编　Dong Weijiang　董炜疆

副主编　Yang Pengbo　杨蓬勃　　Feng Gaifeng　冯改丰
　　　　Jin Hui　靳　辉

编　者　（按姓氏笔画排序）
　　　　Feng Gaifeng　冯改丰　　Sun Tianze　孙天泽
　　　　Li Yueying　李月英　　Yang Weina　杨维娜
　　　　Yang Pengbo　杨蓬勃　　Jia Ning　贾　宁
　　　　Dong Weijiang　董炜疆　　Jin Hui　靳　辉

西安交通大学出版社
XI'AN JIAOTONG UNIVERSITY PRESS

国家一级出版社
全国百佳图书出版单位

图书在版编目(CIP)数据

局部解剖学学习指导及习题集：Learning Instructions and Exercises of Human Regional Anatomy：英文/董炜疆主编. —西安：西安交通大学出版社，2019.9
ISBN 978 - 7 - 5693 - 1281 - 2

Ⅰ. ①局… Ⅱ. ①董… Ⅲ. ①局部解剖学-英文
Ⅳ. ①R323

中国版本图书馆 CIP 数据核字(2019)第 170813 号

书　　名	Learning Instructions and Exercises of Human Regional Anatomy
主　　编	董炜疆
责任编辑	赵丹青

出版发行	西安交通大学出版社
	（西安市兴庆南路 1 号　邮政编码 710048）
网　　址	http://www.xjtupress.com
电　　话	(029)82668357　82667874(发行中心)
	(029)82668315(总编办)
传　　真	(029)82668280
印　　刷	西安日报社印务中心

开　　本	787mm×1092mm　1/16　印张 11.375　字数 364 千字
版次印次	2019 年 9 月第 1 版　2019 年 9 月第 1 次印刷
书　　号	ISBN 978 - 7 - 5693 - 1281 - 2
定　　价	36.00 元

读者购书、书店添货，如发现印装质量问题，请与本社发行中心联系调换。
订购热线：(029)82665248　(029)82665249
投稿热线：(029)82668803　(029)82668804
读者信箱：med_xjup@163.com

Preface

Regional anatomy is an approach to the anatomic study based on regions, parts, or divisions of the body, emphasizing the relationships of various systemic structures within that area. Mastering regional anatomy requires both practices in class and exercises after class.

For more than 20 years, suffering from the lack of English versions of teaching and exercising materials, international students in our university found it difficult to review regional anatomy before the examination, let alone get good grades. To enable international students to grapple the key knowledge of human anatomy in a relatively short time, teachers in the Department of Human Anatomy and Histology and Embryology elaborated on the plans and requirements, compiled *Learning Instructions and Exercises of Human Regional Anatomy*. It supplements the general courses of regional anatomy, providing guidance to international students, teachers and health workers alike.

This book is compiled according to the human anatomy teaching program and the newest version of *A Textbook of Regional Anatomy*. It is arranged in the same pattern as the textbook, with content divided into chapters and sections. The number and difficulty of questions are varied according to the key points and teaching hours, covering the full content of the textbook. Question types range from simple reciting to comprehension and application, including single choice, double choices, fill in the blanks, brief questions and in-detail questions. Model answers are attached to the end of each chapter, suitable as review reference and a tool to consolidate textbook knowledge.

This book consists of eight chapters: the Head, the Neck, the Upper Limb, the Lower Limb, the Thorax, the Abdomen, the Pelvis and Perineum, the Back and Vertebral Region. Authors for this book are all devoted professors and teachers with years of experience in the teaching of human anatomy. This book is designed for international students majoring in medical sciences and Chinese medical students enrolled in 7 or 8-year programs.

Special thanks to the School of International Education for their funding in the writing and publishing of this book. Thanks to Xi'an Jiaotong University Press and Department of Human Anatomy and Histology and Embryology for their support and help. Thanks to the authors of the books we referred in the compilation of this book. Due to the limitations in our knowledge, omissions and errors can hardly be avoided. We welcome any criticisms and corrections.

CONTENTS

Chapter 1 The Head

Section 1 Introduction

Outline and Objectives

Comprehend

1. The boundaries and divisions of the head.
2. The important surface landmarks of head and face, such as the external occipital protuberance, pterion, supraorbital foramen, infraorbital foramen, mental foramen, angle of mandible, mastoid process, etc.
3. The location, formation and clinical notes of the pterion.

Exercises

Ⅰ. **Single choice（Choose the best answer among the following four answers, and write the corresponding letter in the bracket）**

Which of the following does **not** form the boundaries between head and neck? （   ）

A. Lower border of mandible

B. Angle of mandible

C. Styloid process

D. Mastoid process

Ⅱ. **Double choices（Choose the two best answers among the following answers, and write the corresponding letters in the bracket）**

Which of the following form the boundaries between cranium and face? （   ）

A. Infraorbital margin

B. Zygomatic arch

C. Inferior margin of external acoustic meatus

D. Mastoid process

E. External occipital protuberance

III. Fill the blanks (Fill the most appropriate words and phrases in the blanks)

1. The pterion is formed by the junction of four bones, they are _____ , _____ , _____ and _____ .

2. The head is divided into _____ posterosuperiorly and _____ anteroinferiorly by an imaginary line linking with the _____ , _____ , _____ and _____ .

IV. Answer the questions briefly

1. Describe the boundaries and divisions of the head.

2. Describe the location and perforating structures of the supraorbital, infraorbital and mental foramina.

Section 2   The Face

Outline and Objectives

I. Grasp

1. The characteristics of the skin, superficial fascia and muscles of expression.

2. The course and supply of blood vessels and nerves on superficial of the face, especially the facial artery, facial vein and facial nerve.

3. The features, parts and sheath of the parotid gland; the structures which pierce the parotid gland and their arrangement.

4. The name, location and action of the masticatory muscles; the course, branches and distribution of the maxillary artery and mandibular nerve.

II. Comprehend

1. The arrangement of the facial muscles.

2. The position of the terminal branches of the trigeminal nerve which pierce the passage of the skull and its clinical notes.

3. The projection of the location of the parotid duct.

Exercises

I. Single choice (Choose the best answer among the following four answers, and write the corresponding letter in the bracket)

1. About the muscles of expression, which of the following is right? (   )

   A. They contain facial muscles and masticatory muscles.

   B. They are inserted into the cranial bones.

   C. They are inserted into the skin.

   D. They are supplied by the trigeminal nerve.

2. About the parotid gland, which of the following statements is **wrong**? (   )

   A. It locates anterior to the external acoustic meatus.

   B. The greater auricular nerve innervates the skin over the gland.

   C. It has two parts, the superficial part and deep part.

   D. The parotid duct begins from the posterior border of the gland.

3. The facial artery arises from the (   ).

   A. external carotid artery

   B. internal carotid artery

   C. common carotid artery

   D. aortic arch

4. About the facial vein, which of the following statements is **wrong**? (   )

   A. It begins as the angular vein.

   B. It accompanies the facial artery and lies posterior to it.

   C. Inferior to the mandible, it is joined by the anterior branch of the retromandibular vein.

   D. It drains into the external jugular vein.

5. Which of the following is **not** a branch of facial nerve? (   )

   A. Temporal branch

   B. Cervical branch

   C. Buccal nerve

   D. Zygomatic branch

6. The nerve which supplies the skin of the upper eyelid is (   ).

   A. supraorbital nerve

   B. infraorbital nerve

   C. auriculotemporal nerve

   D. buccal nerve

7. Which of the following does **not** pass through the parotid gland? (   )

   A. Facial nerve

   B. Auriculotemporal nerve

   C. Retromandibular vein

   D. Internal carotid artery

8. Which of the following does **not** belong to the masticatory muscles? (   )

   A. Temporalis

   B. Masseter

   C. Occipitofrontalis

   D. Medial pterygoid

9. Which muscle is inserted to the neck of mandible? (   )

   A. Temporalis

   B. Masseter

    C. Lateral pterygoid

    D. Medial pterygoid

10. Which of the following is **not** a branch of maxillary artery? ( )

    A. Inferior alveolar artery

    B. Middle meningeal artery

    C. Infraorbital artery

    D. Superficial temporal artery

II. Double choices (Choose the two best answers among the following answers, and write the corresponding letters in the bracket)

1. Which structures run with the parotid duct? ( )

    A. Zygomatic branch of facial nerve

    B. Buccal branch of facial nerve

    C. Marginal mandibular branch of facial nerve

    D. Transverse facial vessels

    E. Superficial temporal vessels

2. Which of the following do **not** belong to the muscles of expression? ( )

    A. Orbicularis oris

    B. Masseter

    C. Buccinator

    D. Temporalis

    E. Platysma

3. About the facial vessels, which of the following statements are **wrong**? ( )

    A. Facial artery arises from the external carotid artery.

    B. Facial vein begins as the angular vein.

    C. Facial vein drains into the internal jugular vein.

    D. Facial vein is straighter and deeper than facial artery.

    E. Facial artery always accompanies with the facial vein and facial nerve.

4. The following structures pass through the parotid gland, **except** for ( ).

    A. facial nerve

    B. auriculotemporal nerve

    C. retromandibular vein

    D. internal carotid artery

    E. greater auricular nerve

5. Which of the following belong to the branches of the mandibular nerve? ( )

    A. Supraorbital nerve

    B. Infraorbital nerve

    C. Lingual nerve

    D. Superior alveolar nerve

    E. Inferior alveolar nerve

Ⅲ. Fill the blanks (Fill the most appropriate words and phrases in the blanks)

    1. The structures passing through the parotid gland vertically contain _____ , _____ , _____ and _____ .

    2. The structures passing through the parotid gland transversely are _____ , _____ and _____ .

    3. The facial vein begins as the _____ and drains into the _____ .

    4. The branches of facial nerve which innervate the facial muscles are _____ , _____ , _____ , _____ and _____ .

    5. The branches of the first part of maxillary artery are _____ and _____ .

Ⅳ. Answer the questions briefly

    1. Describe the structures passing through the parotid gland vertically.

    2. Describe the structures passing through the parotid gland transversely.

    3. Describe the course of the parotid duct and its accompanying structures.

    4. Describe the branches of the mandibular nerve.

    5. Describe the masticatory muscles and their innervating nerve.

Ⅴ. Answer the questions in detail

    1. Describe the structures passing through the parotid gland.

    2. Describe the divisions and main branches of the maxillary artery.

Section 3   The Cranium

Outline and Objectives

Ⅰ. Grasp

    1. The layers of fronto-parieto-occipital and temporal regions; the characteristics of each layer of them; the conception of scalp proper.

    2. The communications which are between extracranial and intracranial veins as well as its clinical notes.

    3. The formation and main structures of anterior, middle and posterior cranial fossae.

Ⅱ. Comprehend

    1. The divisions of the skull.

    2. The cerebral dura mater and venous sinus; the location and perforating structures of the cavernous sinus.

Exercises

I. Single choice (Choose the best answer among the following four answers, and write the corresponding letter in the bracket)

1. About the skin of scalp, which of the following is **wrong**? (   )
   A. It is thick and dense.
   B. It consists of hair bulbs, sweat glands and sebaceous gland.
   C. It is liable to bleeding.
   D. It is loosely bound to the superficial fascia.

2. Which of the following is **not** the characteristic of the subaponeurotic loose connective tissue? (   )
   A. It lies between the scalp proper and the pericranium.
   B. Through this layer, scalp proper is loosely bound to the pericranium.
   C. The blood vessels and nerves of calva are mainly distributed in this layer.
   D. Blood may spread in this space during trauma.

3. The scalp proper contains the following structures, **except** for (   ).
   A. skin
   B. superficial fascia
   C. epicranial aponeurosis
   D. subaponeurotic loose connective tissue

4. The blood vessels and nerves of calvaria are mainly distributed in (   ).
   A. skin
   B. superficial fascia
   C. epicranial aponeurosis
   D. subaponeurotic loose connective tissue

5. About the temporal fascia, which of the following is **wrong**? (   )
   A. It is dense fascia.
   B. It lies beneath the temporalis.
   C. It is separated into two layers by some fatty tissue.
   D. Deep layer is attached to the upper border and inner surface of zygomatic arch.

6. Which of the following does **not** pass through the superior orbital fissure? (   )
   A. Oculomotor nerve
   B. Trochlear nerve
   C. Ophthalmic nerve
   D. Maxillary nerve

7. Which bone does **not** form the anterior cranial fossa? (   )
   A. Frontal bone
   B. Sphenoid bone
   C. Temporal bone
   D. Ethmoid bone

8. The structure which lies in the middle cranial fossa is (   ).

   A. cribriform foramina

   B. hypophysial fossa

   C. jugular foramen

   D. inferior orbital fissure

9. The pterion is formed by the following bones, **except** for (   ).

   A. frontal bone

   B. parietal bone

   C. temporal bone

   D. occipital bone

10. About the cerebral dura mater, which of the following is **wrong**? (   )

   A. It has two layers.

   B. It forms the venous sinuses.

   C. Two layers are loosely united.

   D. The outer layer is continuous with the pericranium.

Ⅱ. **Double choices (Choose the two best answers among the following answers, and write the corresponding letters in the bracket)**

1. The structures pass through the medial side of the cavernous sinus are (   ).

   A. internal carotid artery

   B. external carotid artery

   C. oculomotor nerve

   D. trochlear nerve

   E. abducent nerve

2. About the temporalis, which of the following are right? (   )

   A. It belongs to the facial muscles.

   B. It arises from the zygomatic arch.

   C. It is inserted into the coronoid process of mandible.

   D. It lies beneath the temporal fascia.

   E. It is innervated by the branch of maxillary nerve.

3. The following structures pass through the lateral wall of the cavernous sinus, **except** for (   ).

   A. optic nerve

   B. ophthalmic nerve

   C. oculomotor nerve

   D. trochlear nerve

   E. abducent nerve

4. The venous sinuses which lie in the upper and lower margins of the cerebral falx are
   (   ).
   A. superior sagittal sinus
   B. inferior sagittal sinus
   C. straight sinus
   D. transverse sinus
   E. sigmoid sinus
5. The following nerves pass through the jugular foramen, **except** for (   ).
   A. facial nerve
   B. trigeminal nerve
   C. glossopharyngeal nerve
   D. vagus nerve
   E. accessory nerve

Ⅲ. Fill the blanks (Fill the most appropriate words and phrases in the blanks)

1. The scalp proper is formed by _____ , _____ and _____ .
2. From superficial to deep, the layers of temporal region are _____ , _____ ,
   _____ , _____ and _____ .
3. From superficial to deep, the layers of front-oparieto-occipital region are _____ ,
   _____ , _____ , _____ and _____ .
4. The structures passing through the lateral wall of the cavernous sinus are _____ ,
   _____ , _____ and _____ .
5. The structures passing through the medial wall of the cavernous sinus are _____
   and _____ .

Ⅳ. Answer the questions briefly

1. Describe the layers of fronto-parieto-occipital region.
2. Describe the layers of temporal region.
3. Describe the location and perforating structures of cavernous sinus.
4. Describe the structures formed by the cerebral dura mater.

Ⅴ. Answer the questions in detail

Describe the layers and characteristics of the fronto-parieto-occipital region.

Chapter 2   The Neck

Section 1   Introduction

Outline and Objectives

Comprehend

1. The boundaries and divisions of the neck.
2. The principal surface landmarks and projections of the neck.
3. The clinical notes of the cricoid cartilage.

Exercises

Ⅰ. **Single choice（Choose the best answer among the following four answers, and write the corresponding letter in the bracket）**

1. Which of the following does **not** form the boundaries between head and neck? (   )
    A. Upper border of mandible
    B. Angle of mandible
    C. Mastoid process
    D. External occipital protuberance

2. The following structures form the inferior boundaries of the neck, **except** for (   ).
    A. upper border of sternum
    B. clavicle
    C. upper border of scapula
    D. spine of the 7th cervical vertebra

3. The neck can be divided into the nape and side of neck by (   ).
    A. anterior margin of sternocleidomastoid
    B. posterior margin of sternocleidomastoid
    C. anterior margin of trapezius
    D. posterior margin of trapezius

4. The side of neck can be subdivided into three regions by (   ).
    A. trapezius
    B. sternocleidomastoid
    C. hyoid bone
    D. thyroid cartilage

5. Which of the following belongs to the suprahyoid region? (   )

A. Carotid triangle

B. Muscular triangle

C. Occipital triangle

D. Submental triangle

6. Which of the following belongs to the infrahyoid region? (   )

A. Carotid triangle

B. Submandibular triangle

C. Occipital triangle

D. Submental triangle

7. The level of cricoid cartilage corresponds to the (   ).

A. junction of the larynx with trachea

B. junction of the oral cavity with pharynx

C. end of common carotid artery

D. 4th cervical vertebra

8. The upper border of thyroid cartilage corresponds to the beginning of (   ).

A. common carotid artery

B. internal carotid artery

C. internal jugular vein

D. external jugular vein

9. About the hyoid bone, which of the following is **wrong**? (   )

A. It lies opposite to the third cervical vertebra.

B. Its greater horn can be felt on both sides of the body.

C. Its lesser horn can be felt on both sides of the body.

D. It is the landmark to look for the lingual artery.

10. The surface projection of external jugular vein is on the line between (   ).

A. angle of mandible and midpoint of clavicle

B. mastoid process and midpoint of clavicle

C. angle of mandible and sternoclavicular joint

D. mastoid process and sternoclavicular joint

II. Double choices (Choose the two best answers among the following answers, and write the corresponding letters in the bracket)

1. Which of the following do **not** form the boundaries of submandibular triangle? (   )

A. Median line of the neck

B. Anterior belly of digastric

C. Posterior belly of digastric

D. Body of hyoid bone

E. Lower border of mandible

2. The submental triangle is bounded by the following structures, **except** for (   ).

A. left anterior belly of digastric

B. right anterior belly of digastric

C. posterior belly of digastric

D. body of hyoid bone

E. lower border of mandible

3. The carotid triangle is bounded by the following structures, **except** for (   ).

A. anterior margin of sternocleidomastoid

B. posterior margin of sternocleidomastoid

C. anterior belly of digastric

D. posterior belly of digastric

E. superior belly of omohyoid

4. Which of the following do **not** form the boundaries of muscular triangle? (   )

A. Anterior margin of sternocleidomastoid

B. Posterior margin of sternocleidomastoid

C. Superior belly of omohyoid

D. Inferior belly of omohyoid

E. Median line of the neck

5. The lateral region of the neck contains (   ).

A. occipital triangle

B. carotid triangle

C. muscular triangle

D. supraclavicular fossa

E. submandibular triangle

Ⅲ. Fill the blanks (Fill the most appropriate words and phrases in the blanks)

1. The side of neck can be subdivided into three regions _____ , _____ and _____ .

2. The suprahyoid region contains _____ and _____ .

3. The infrahyoid region contains _____ and _____ .

4. The boundaries of carotid triangle are _____ , _____ and _____ .

5. The occipital triangle is enclosed by _____ , _____ and _____ .

Ⅳ. Answer the questions briefly

1. The boundaries of the muscular triangle.

2. The boundaries of the carotid triangle.

3. The boundaries of the submandibular triangle.

Ⅴ. Answer the questions in detail

Describe the boundaries and divisions of the neck.

Section 2   The Superficial Structures and Cervical Fascia

Outline and Objectives

Ⅰ. Grasp

1. The distribution of the superficial veins and cutaneous nerves.
2. The layers of the cervical fascia and the formations of each of them.

Ⅱ. Comprehend

1. The location and innervating nerve of platysma.
2. The fascial spaces of the neck and their contents, especially the suprasternal space, pretracheal space and submandibular space.

Exercises

Ⅰ. Single choice (Choose the best answer among the following four answers, and write the corresponding letter in the bracket)

1. The platysma is innervated by (   ).
    A. vagus nerve
    B. facial nerve
    C. trigeminal nerve
    D. accessory nerve
2. Which of the following belongs to the superficial vein of the neck? (   )
    A. Facial vein
    B. Internal jugular vein
    C. Anterior jugular vein
    D. Lingual vein
3. Which nerve does **not** lie in the neck? (   )
    A. Cervical branch of facial nerve
    B. Buccal branch of facial nerve
    C. Transverse nerve of neck
    D. Greater auricular nerve
4. The cutaneous branches of cervical plexus piece the deep fascia at (   ).
    A. midpoint of the anterior border of sternocleidomastoid
    B. midpoint of the posterior border of sternocleidomastoid
    C. midpoint of the anterior border of trapezius
    D. midpoint of the posterior border of trapezius

5. Which of the following belongs to the cutaneous branches of cervical plexus? (   )

    A. Greater occipital nerve

    B. Supraclavicular nerve

    C. Transverse nerve of neck

    D. Greater auricular nerve

6. From superficial to deep, the cervical fasciae are (   ).

    A. investing fascia, prevertebral fascia, visceral fascia

    B. investing fascia, visceral fascia, prevertebral fascia

    C. visceral fascia, investing fascia, prevertebral fascia

    D. visceral fascia, prevertebral fascia, investing fascia

7. Which of the following is **not** enclosed by the investing fascia? (   )

    A. Parotid gland

    B. Sublingual gland

    C. Sternocleidomastoid

    D. Trapezius

8. The following structures are formed by the investing fascia, **except** for (   ).

    A. suprasternal space

    B. submandibular space

    C. pretracheal space

    D. sheath of parotid gland

9. The pretracheal fascia encloses (   ).

    A. parotid gland

    B. sublingual gland

    C. submandibular gland

    D. thyroid gland

10. The prevertebral fascia covers the following structures, **except** for (   ).

    A. scalenus anterior

    B. levator scapula

    C. common carotid artery

    D. brachial plexus

11. Which of the following does **not** lie in the carotid sheath? (   )

    A. Internal jugular vein

    B. External jugular vein

    C. Common carotid artery

    D. Internal carotid artery

12. Which of the following does **not** lie in the suprasternal space? (   )

    A. Anterior jugular vein

    B. External jugular vein

     C. Jugular venous arch

     D. Sternal head of sternocleidomastoid

13. About the external jugular vein, which of the following is **not** true? (   )

     A. It is a superficial vein in the neck.

     B. It runs downwards on the surface of sternocleidomastoid.

     C. The anterior division of retromandibular vein drains to it.

     D. The posterior auricular vein drains to it.

14. The axillary sheath encloses the following structures, **except** for (   ).

     A. axillary artery

     B. axillary vein

     C. cervical plexus

     D. brachial plexus

15. Which of the following does **not** lie in the pretracheal space? (   )

     A. Inferior thyroid vein

     B. Lowest thyroid artery

     C. Brachiocephalic trunk

     D. Right brachiocephalic vein

II. Double choices (Choose the two best answers among the following answers, and write the corresponding letters in the bracket)

1. About the platysma, which of the following are **not** true? (   )

     A. It belongs to the muscles of expression.

     B. It arises from the fasciae of pectoralis minor and deltoid.

     C. It is inserted into the skin of the lower part of face.

     D. It lies in the superficial fascia of neck.

     E. It is innervated by the branch of cervical plexus.

2. Which of the muscles are enclosed by enveloping fascia? (   )

     A. Platysma

     B. Sternocleidomastoid

     C. Omohyoid

     D. Trapezius

     E. Digastric

3. Which of the glands are enclosed by investing fascia? (   )

     A. Parotid gland

     B. Sublingual gland

     C. Submandibular gland

     D. Thyroid gland

     E. Parathyroid gland

4. Which of the following structures lie in the pretracheal space? (   )

    A. Middle thyroid vein

    B. inferior thyroid artery

    C. Brachiocephalic trunk

    D. Lowest thyroid artery

    E. Right brachiocephalic vein

5. Which of the following do **not** belong to the superficial structures of the neck? (   )

    A. Platysma

    B. Digastric

    C. Anterior jugular vein

    D. External jugular vein

    E. External carotid artery

III. Fill the blanks (Fill the most appropriate words and phrases in the blanks)

1. The investing fascia divides into two layers to encloses _____ and _____ two muscles, _____ and _____ two glands.

2. The cervical fascia can be divided into three layers, they are _____, _____ and _____.

3. The external jugular vein arises from the union of _____ and _____, and it ends mainly in _____.

4. The axillary sheath surrounds the _____, _____ and _____.

5. The carotid sheath encloses the _____, _____, _____ and _____.

IV. Answer the questions briefly

1. The attachment and formation of the enveloping fascia.

2. The attachment and formation of the prevertebral fascia.

3. The location and contents of the carotid sheath.

4. The formation and contents of the suprasternal space.

5. The formation and contents of the pretracheal space.

V. Answer the questions in detail

1. Describe the layers of cervical fascia and their attachment and formations.

2. Describe the superficial nerves of the neck and their distribution.

Section 3   The Anterior Region of the Neck

Outline and Objectives

I. Grasp

1. The boundaries and contents of the carotid triangle.

    2. The boundaries and contents of the muscular triangle.

    3. The boundaries and contents of the submandibular triangle.

    3. The features, location, relationship, coverings, blood vessels and nerves of the thyroid gland.

    4. The relationship of the cervical part of trachea.

Ⅱ. Comprehend

    1. The boundaries and contents of the submental triangle.

    2. The cervical part of esophagus.

Exercises

Ⅰ. Single choice (Choose the best answer among the following four answers, and write the corresponding letter in the bracket)

    1. Which of the following does **not** form the boundaries of submandibular triangle? (　　)

        A. Lower border of mandible

        B. Anterior belly of digastric

        C. Posterior belly of digastric

        D. Anterior border of sternocleidomastoid

    2. Which of the following does **not** belong to the contents of submandibular triangle? (　　)

        A. Submandibular gland

        B. Facial artery

        C. Vagus nerve

        D. Hypoglossal nerve

    3. About the submandibular gland, which of the following is **not** true? (　　)

        A. It has a greater superficial part and a smaller deep part.

        B. The submandibular duct arises from the superficial part.

        C. It is covered by the skin, superficial fascia, platysma and enveloping fascia.

        D. The hypoglossal nerve runs below the gland and duct.

    4. The secretion of submandibular and sublingual glands is innervated by (　　).

        A. lingual nerve

        B. hypoglossal nerve

        C. facial nerve

        D. trigeminal nerve

    5. About the submental triangle, which of the following is **wrong**? (　　)

        A. It is enclosed by hyoid bone, left and right superior bellies of digastric.

        B. The mylohyoid forms its floor.

        C. The enveloping fascia forms its roof.

        D. There are submental lymph nodes and facial vessels in this triangle.

6. Which of the following does **not** form the boundaries of carotid triangle? (   )

    A. Anterior margin of sternocleidomastoid

    B. Anterior belly of digastric

    C. Posterior belly of digastric

    D. Superior belly of omohyoid

7. Internal jugular vein receives the blood from the following veins, **except** for (   ).

    A. facial vein

    B. lingual vein

    C. posterior auricular vein

    D. middle thyroid vein

8. Which of the following is **not** the branch of external carotid artery? (   )

    A. Facial artery

    B. Occipital artery

    C. Lingual artery

    D. Inferior thyroid artery

9. The ansa cervicalis is formed by the union of 2nd, 3rd cervical nerves and the branch of (   ).

    A. facial nerve

    B. vagus nerve

    C. lingual nerve

    D. hypoglossal nerve

10. Which of the following does **not** lie in the carotid triangle? (   )

    A. Common carotid artery

    B. Internal jugular vein

    C. Hypoglossal nerve

    D. Lingual nerve

11. Which of the following does **not** form the boundaries of muscular triangle? (   )

    A. Anterior margin of sternocleidomastoid

    B. Superior belly of omohyoid

    C. Posterior belly of digastric

    D. Median line of the neck

12. Which of the following does **not** lie in the muscular triangle? (   )

    A. Thyroid gland

    B. Sternothyroid

    C. Submandibular gland

    D. Cervical part of esophagus

13. About the relationship of thyroid gland, which of the following is **wrong**? (   )

    A. The isthmus extends across the 2nd – 4th rings of trachea.

    B. The skin, superficial fascia, enveloping fascia, suprahyoid muscles and the pre-tracheal fasciais in front of the gland.

    C. The posteromedial aspect of lateral lobe contacts with the larynx, trachea, pharynx, esophagus and recurrent laryngeal nerve.

    D. Lateral to the lateral lobes there are the carotid sheath and the sympathetic trunk.

14. About the thyroid arteries, which of the following is **wrong**? (　　)

    A. The superior thyroid artery accompanies with the superior laryngeal nerve.

    B. The inferior thyroid artery accompanies with the recurrent laryngeal nerve.

    C. The lowest thyroid artery lies in the pretracheal space.

    D. All of the thyroid arteries arise from the external carotid artery.

15. Which of the following drains into the brachiocephalic vein? (　　)

    A. Superior thyroid vein

    B. Middle thyroid vein

    C. Inferior thyroid vein

    D. All of above

Ⅱ. Double choices (Choose the two best answers among the following answers, and write the corresponding letters in the bracket)

1. About the vagus nerve, which of the following are **wrong**? (　　)

    A. It leaves the skull through jugular foramen.

    B. It lies in the posterior part of the carotid sheath.

    C. The cricothyroid is innervated by the superior laryngeal nerve.

    D. All the mucous membrane of larynx is innervated by recurrent laryngeal nerve.

    E. Right recurrent laryngeal nerve hooks around the aortic arch.

2. About the thyroid gland, which of the following are right? (　　)

    A. It lies in muscular triangle.

    B. It consists of one lateral lobe and one isthmus.

    C. It is enclosed by two coverings.

    D. The outer covering is thyroid sheath and formed by pretracheal fascia.

    E. The inner covering is fibrous capsule and formed by prevertebral fascia.

3. The anterior border of sternocleidomastoid forms the boundary of (　　).

    A. carotid triangle

    B. submental triangle

    C. muscular triangle

    D. submandibular triangle

    E. occipital triangle

4. Which of the following about parathyroid glands are **wrong**? (　　)

    A. There are two pairs of parathyroid glands.

    B. They lie along the posterior border of the isthmus of thyroid gland.

    C. They are enclosed by fibrous capsule of thyroid gland.

    D. They are located between thyroid sheath and fibrous capsule of thyroid gland.

    E. The superior parathyroid glands are more constant in position.

5. Which of the muscles are innervated by ansa cervicalis? (   )

   A. Sternothyroid

   B. Omohyoid

   C. Platysma

   D. Digastric

   E. Sternocleidomastoid

Ⅲ. **Fill the blanks （Fill the most appropriate words and phrases in the blanks）**

   1. The anterior region of the neck is divided by hyoid bone into _____ and _____ two parts.

   2. The carotid triangle is enclosed by _____ , _____ and _____ .

   3. The infrahyoid muscles consist of _____ , _____ , _____ and _____ ____ .

   4. The sheath of submandibular gland is formed by _____ , and the thyroid sheath is formed by _____ .

   5. The superior thyroid artery arises from _____ , the inferior thyroid artery arises from _____ .

   6. Left recurrent laryngeal nerve hooks around _____ , right recurrent laryngeal nerve hooks around _____ .

Ⅳ. **Answer the questions briefly**

   1. The boundaries and contents of submandibular triangle.

   2. The boundaries and contents of carotid triangle.

   3. The boundaries and contents of muscular triangle.

   4. The anterior relationship of the cervical part of trachea.

Ⅴ. **Answer the questions in detail**

   1. Describe the location, relationship and coverings of thyroid gland.

   2. Describe the blood vessels of thyroid gland and the considerations for thyroid surgery.

Section 4   The Sternocleidomastoid Region of the Neck

Outline and Objectives

Ⅰ. **Grasp**

   1. The superficial structures of the sternocleidomastoid region.

   2. The deep structures of the sternocleidomastoid region.

   3. The formation, location and function of the ansa cervicalis.

   4. The contents and their relationship of the carotid sheath.

5. The branches and distributions of the cervical plexus, the landmark for local anesthesia for cervical plexus.

II. Comprehend

The sympathetic trunk in the neck.

Exercises

I. Single choice (Choose the best answer among the following four answers, and write the corresponding letter in the bracket)

1. Which of the following does **not** lie in the sternocleidomastoid region? (   )

   A. Ansa cervicalis

   B. Carotid sheath

   C. Cervical plexus

   D. Submandibular gland

2. The landmark for local anesthesia of cervical plexus is (   ).

   A. midpoint of the anterior border of sternocleidomastoid

   B. midpoint of the posterior border of sternocleidomastoid

   C. midpoint of the anterior border of trapezius

   D. midpoint of the posterior border of trapezius

3. The following structures lie in front of the carotid sheath, **except** for (   ).

   A. mylohyoid

   B. sternocleidomastoid

   C. sternohyoid

   D. omohyoid

4. Above the upper border of thyroid cartilage, which of the following does **not** in the carotid sheath? (   )

   A. Common carotid artery

   B. Internal carotid artery

   C. Internal jugular vein

   D. Vagus nerve

5. Below the upper border of thyroid cartilage, which of the following does **not** in the carotid sheath? (   )

   A. Common carotid artery

   B. Internal carotid artery

   C. Internal jugular vein

   D. Vagus nerve

6. The ansa cervicalis innervates the following muscles, **except** for (   ).

   A. sternothyroid

   B. sternocleidomastoid

C. sternohyoid

D. omohyoid

7. The cervical plexus is formed by (   ).

A. anterior branches of $C_1 - C_4$

B. anterior branches of $C_5 - C_8$

C. posterior branches of $C_1 - C_4$

D. posterior branches of $C_5 - C_8$

8. The sympathetic trunk in the neck is covered by (   ).

A. enveloping fascia

B. pretracheal fascia

C. prevertebral fascia

D. none of them

II . Double choices (Choose the two best answers among the following answers, and write the corresponding letters in the bracket)

1. Which of the following do **not** lie in the carotid sheath? (   )

A. Vagus nerve

B. Internal carotid artery

C. Internal jugular vein

D. External jugular vein

E. Hypoglossal nerve

2. About the ansa cervicalis, which of the following are **wrong**? (   )

A. It is formed by two roots.

B. The upper root arises from the lingual nerve.

C. The lower root arises from the 2nd and 3rd cervical nerves.

D. It lies on the anterior surface of carotid sheath.

E. It innervates the suprahyoid muscles.

3. Which of the nerves belong to the branches of cervical plexus? (   )

A. Phrenic nerve

B. Recurrent laryngeal nerve

C. Long thoracic nerve

D. Greater auricular nerve

E. Greater occipital nerve

4. About the sympathetic trunk in the neck, which of the following are right? (   )

A. It lies on the surface of the prevertebral fascia.

B. It consists of three ganglia.

C. The superior cervical ganglion is very small.

D. The middle cervical ganglion is the largest one.

E. The inferior cervical ganglion usually unites with the first thoracic ganglion.

5. Which of the following lie medial to the carotid sheath? (   )

A. Sympathetic trunk

B. Ansa cervicalis

C. Larynx

D. Sternothyroid

E. Recurrent laryngeal nerve

III. Fill the blanks (Fill the most appropriate words and phrases in the blanks)

1. The cervical plexus is formed by the anterior branches of the _____.

2. The upper root of ansa cervicalis arises from _____, and the lower root arises from _____.

3. The muscles innervated by ansa cervicalis are _____, _____ and _____.

4. The contents of the carotid sheath are _____, _____, _____ and _____.

5. The superficial branches of cervical plexus are _____, _____, _____ and _____.

6. Left recurrent laryngeal nerve hooks around _____, right recurrent laryngeal nerve hooks around _____.

IV. Answer the questions briefly

1. The formation and distribution of the ansa cervicalis.

2. The contents of carotid sheath.

3. The formation, location and main branches of cervical plexus.

V. Answer the questions in detail

Describe the location, relationship and contents of carotid sheath.

Section 5   The Lateral Region of the Neck

Outline and Objectives

Comprehend

1. The boundaries and contents of the occipital triangle.

2. The boundaries and contents of the supraclavicular fossa.

3. The boundaries and contents of the scalene fissure.

4. The structures surround the scalenus anterior and their relationship.

5. The branches and distributions of the subclavian artery.

6. The boundaries and contents of the triangle of vertebral artery.

Exercises

I . Single choice (Choose the best answer among the following four answers, and write the corresponding letter in the bracket)

1. Which one does **not** form the boundaries of the lateral region of neck? (   )

    A. Anterior border of sternocleidomastoid

    B. Posterior border of sternocleidomastoid

    C. Anterior border of trapezius

    D. Middle third of clavicle

2. The boundaries of occipital triangle are as following, **except** for (   ).

    A. posterior border of sternocleidomastoid

    B. inferior belly of omohyoid

    C. anterior border of trapezius

    D. middle third of clavicle

3. The boundaries of greater supraclavicular fossa are as following, **except** for (   ).

    A. posterior border of sternocleidomastoid

    B. inferior belly of omohyoid

    C. anterior border of trapezius

    D. middle third of clavicle

4. Which one does **not** lie in the occipital triangle? (   )

    A. External branch of accessory nerve

    B. Vagus nerve

    C. Lateral jugular lymph node

    D. Lesser occipital nerve

5. The cutaneous branches of cervical plexus piece the deep fascia at (   ).

    A. midpoint of the anterior border of sternocleidomastoid

    B. midpoint of the posterior border of sternocleidomastoid

    C. midpoint of the anterior border of trapezius

    D. midpoint of the posterior border of trapezius

6. The scalene fissure lies between (   ).

    A. scalenus anterior and scalenus medius

    B. scalenus medius and scalenus posterior

    C. scalenus posterior and levator scapula

    D. scalenus anterior and sternocleidomastoid

7. Which one transmits the scalene fissure? (   )

    A. Common carotid artery

    B. External jugular vein

    C. Subclavian artery

    D. Subclavian vein

8. Which of the following lies in front of the scalenus anterior? (   )

    A. Subclavian artery

    B. Brachial plexus

    C. Phrenic nerve

    D. Hypoglossal nerve

9. About the subclavian artery, which of the following is true? (   )

    A. Right subclavian artery arises from aortic arch.

    B. Left subclavian artery arises from brachiocephalic trunk.

    C. It arches laterally in the root of neck behind the cupula of pleura.

    D. It ends at the lateral border of the first rib.

10. The subclavian artery is divided into three parts by (   ).

    A. scalenus anterior

    B. scalenus medius

    C. scalenus posterior

    D. sternocleidomastoid

11. Which of the following does **not** belong to the branches of the subclavian artery? (   )

    A. Vertebral artery

    B. Thyrocervical trunk

    C. Superior thyroid artery

    D. Internal thoracic artery

12. About the subclavian vein, which of the following is **wrong**? (   )

    A. It begins at the lateral border of the first rib.

    B. It ends at the medial border of the scalenus anterior.

    C. It transmits the scalene fissure.

    D. It unites with the internal jugular vein to form brachiocephalic vein.

13. The thoracic duct opens into (   ).

    A. left external jugular vein

    B. right external jugular vein

    C. left venous angle

    D. right venous angle

14. The Virchow's lymph node lies in (   ).

    A. left venous angle

    B. right venous angle

    C. both sides of internal jugular vein

    D. root of external jugular vein

Ⅱ. **Double choices (Choose the two best answers among the following answers, and write the corresponding letters in the bracket)**

    1. The arteries arising from the subclavian artery directly are (   ).

    A. vertebral artery

    B. thyrocervical trunk

    C. superior thyroid artery

    D. inferior thyroid artery

    E. suprascapular artery

2. The lateral region of the neck contains (　　).

    A. submandibular triangle

    B. carotid triangle

    C. occipital triangle

    D. muscular triangle

    E. greater supraclavicular fossa

3. The structures transmitting the scalene fissure are (　　).

    A. cervical plexus

    B. external jugular vein

    C. subclavian artery

    D. subclavian vein

    E. brachial plexus

4. Which of the following belong to the branches of supraclavicular part of brachial plexus? (　　)

    A. Ulnar nerve

    B. Dorsal scapular nerve

    C. Median nerve

    D. Subscapular nerve

    E. Long thoracic nerve

5. The muscles innervated by accessory nerve are (　　).

    A. sternohyoid

    B. sternocleidomastoid

    C. digastric

    D. trapezius

    E. platysma

6. The following structures lie in front of the scalenus anterior, **except** for (　　).

    A. subclavian artery

    B. subclavian vein

    C. apex of lung

    D. phrenic nerve

    E. transverse cervical artery

7. About the phrenic nerve, which of the following are **wrong**? (　　)

    A. It is the branch of cervical plexus.

    B. It lies behind thescalenus anterior.

      C. It is deep to the prevertebral fascia.

      D. It gives off the recurrent laryngeal nerve.

      E. It innervates the sternocleidomastoid and trapezius.

  8. About the cupula of pleura, which of the following are right? (   )

      A. It belongs to the visceral pleura.

      B. It covers the base of the lung.

      C. It extends to the root of neck for 2. 5 cm above the clavicle.

      D. Subclavian artery and its branches lie in front of it.

      E. Scalenus anterior lies behind of it.

Ⅲ. Fill the blanks (Fill the most appropriate words and phrases in the blanks)

  1. The lateral region of the neck contains _____ and _____ two parts, and they are separated by _____.

  2. The structures transmitting the scalene fissure are _____ and _____.

  3. The subclavian artery arises from _____ (left) and _____ (right), respectively, and ends at the lateral border of the _____.

  4. The branches of the first part of subclavian artery are _____, _____, _____ and _____.

  5. The branches of the supraclavicular part of brachial plexus are _____, _____ and _____.

  6. Venous angle lies at the junction of _____ and _____, _____ opens into the left venous angle, _____ opens into the right venous angle.

Ⅳ. Answer the questions briefly

  1. The divisions and main branches of the subclavian artery.

  2. The boundaries and contents of the occipital triangle.

  3. The course in lateral region of neck and innervating muscles of the accessory nerve.

  4. The formation and transmitting structures of the scalene fissure.

  5. The formation and receptive structures of the venous angle.

  6. The boundaries and contents of the triangle of vertebral artery.

Ⅴ. Answer the questions in detail

  1. Describe the location and relationship of the cupula of pleura.

  2. Describe the origin, insertion and relationship of the scalenus anterior.

Chapter 3 The Upper Limb

Section 1 Introduction

Outline and Objectives

I. Grasp

1. The origin, course and drainage of the cephalic, basilic and median cubital veins, as well as the clinic significance of them.
2. The concept of the carrying angle and its clinic.

II. Comprehend

1. The boundaries and partitions of the upper limb.
2. The important surface landmarks. Such as acromion, coracoid process, deltoid tuberosity, biceps brachii, olecranon, medial and lateral epicondyle of humerus, flexor tendons, anatomical snuffbox, styloid processes of ulna and radius, etc.
3. The surface projections. For example, the brachial artery, median nerve, ulnar nerve, and so on.
4. The position and drainage of the superficial lymph nodes.

Exercises

I. Single choice (Choose the best answer among the following four answers, and write the corresponding letter in the bracket)

1. About the way of measuring and examining upper limbs, the **wrong** one is (   ).
   A. using anatomical markers
   B. using bony processes
   C. affected limb is examined and recorded only
   D. bilateral control examination

2. About the description of axis and carrying angle of upper limb, which description is **wrong**? (   )
   A. The axis of the upper limb is the connection of the center of head of humerus, the capitulum of humerus and the head of ulna.
   B. The carrying angle is about 10 – 15 degrees normally.

C. Cubitus valgus with carrying angle is greater than 15 degrees.

D. Cubitus varus with carrying angle is less than 10 degrees.

II. Fill the blanks (Fill the most appropriate words and phrases in the blanks)

1. The subdivisions of shoulder area are _____ , _____ and _____ .

2. The main superficial veins of upper limb contain _____ , _____ and _____ .

Section 2   The Shoulder

Outline and Objectives

I. Grasp

1. The position, formation (apex, base, and walls) and contents of the axilla.

2. The positions and boundaries of the triangular (trilateral) and quadrangular (quadrilateral) spaces, and the structures passing through these spaces.

3. The formation, location and main branches (such as median, radial, ulnar, axillary, musculocutaneous, long thoracic and thoracodorsal nerves) of the brachial plexus; the start-stop, segments, branches and distribution of the axillary artery.

4. The groups, arrangements and drainages of the axillary lymph nodes.

5. The name, position, function and nerve supplying of the muscles of shoulder; the origin, insertion and actions of the deltoid.

II. Comprehend

1. The boundary, division and the characteristics of the superficial structures of the shoulder region.

2. The formation and clinical significance of the arterial rete around shoulder.

3. The structures passing through the clavipectoral fascia.

4. The general situation and the distribution of the cutaneousnerves of shoulder.

Exercises

I. Single choice (Choose the best answer among the following four answers, and write the corresponding letter in the bracket)

1. The structure that does **not** constitute the anterior wall of the axilla is (   ).

A. pectoralis major

B. pectoralis minor

C. subclavius and clavipectoral fascia

D. coracobrachialis

2. The structure passing through the trilateral space is (   ).

A. subscapular nerve

B. thoracodorsal nerve

C. scapular circumflex vessels

D. axillary nerve

3. The structure that does **not** pass through the quadrilateral space is (   ).

A. axillary nerve

B. anterior humeral circumflex vessels

C. posterior humeral circumflex vessels

D. scapular circumflex vessels

4. The axillary lymph nodes arranged along the lateral thoracic vessels are (   ).

A. apical lymph nodes

B. central lymph nodes

C. pectoral lymph nodes

D. subscapular lymph nodes

5. The nerve which innervates anterior serratus accompanying with the lateral thoracic artery is (   ).

A. long thoracic nerve

B. subscapular nerve

C. intercostal nerve

D. thoracodorsal nerve

6. The muscles formed posterior wall of axilla do **not** contain (   ).

A. subscapularis

B. teres major

C. latissimus dorsi

D. infraspinatus

7. The following structures pass through the clavipectoral fascia, **except** (   ).

A. lateral thoracic nerve

B. medial thoracic nerve

C. cephalic vein

D. thoracoacromial vessels

8. Which of the following belongs to the branch of first segment of the axillary? (   )

A. Anterior circumflex humeral artery

B. Posterior circumflex humeral artery

C. Lateral thoracic artery

D. Superior thoracic artery

9. The base of axilla is formed by structures as follows, **except** (   ).

A. skin

B. superficial fascia

C. clavipectoral fascia

D. axillary fascia

10. The axillary lymph nodes arranged along proximal part of the axillary vein is (　　).
    A. pectoral lymph node
    B. subscapular lymph node
    C. apical lymph node
    D. lateral lymph node

11. The axillary lymph nodes arranged along the subscapular vessels is (　　).
    A. apical lymph node
    B. pectoral lymph node
    C. lateral lymph node
    D. subscapular lymph node

12. The structure between the trilateral space and the quadrilateral space is (　　).
    A. long head of biceps brachii
    B. short head of biceps brachii
    C. long head of triceps brachii
    D. latissimus dorsi

Ⅱ. Double choices(Choose the two best answers among the following answers, and write the corresponding letters in the bracket)

1. The branches that do **not** belong to the third segment of the axillary artery are (　　).
    A. thoracoacromial artery
    B. subscapular artery
    C. posterior circumflex brachial artery
    D. anterior circumflex brachial artery
    E. superior thoracic artery

2. When axillary lymph nodes are removed during radical mastectomy of breast cancer, which nerves should be avoiding to injure? (　　)
    A. subscapular nerve
    B. lateral thoracic nerve
    C. long thoracic nerve
    D. dorsothoracic nerve
    E. axillary nerve

3. Regarding the posterior wall of the axilla, which descriptions are **incorrect**? (　　)
    A. The lateral boundary of the trilateral foramen is the long head of triceps brachii.
    B. The lateral boundary of the quadrilateral foramen is the long head of triceps brachii.
    C. It makes up of teres major, latissimus dorsi, subscapularis and scapula.
    D. Trilateral foramen transmits the subscapular artery.
    E. The lower boundary of the quadrilateral foramen is the major teres.

4. Which of the following are **not** main constituents of scapular arterial network? (　　)
    A. Suprascapular artery
    B. Dorsal scapular artery

C. Circumflex scapular artery

D. Anterior circumflex brachial artery

E. Posterior circumflex brachial artery

5. Which of the following structures do **not** participate in the shoulder sleeves? (   )

A. Tendon of teres major

B. Tendon of teres minor

C. Tendon of infraspinatus

D. Tendon of supraspinatus

E. Tendon of latissimus dorsi

III. Fill the blanks (**Fill the most appropriate words and phrases in the blanks**)

1. The apexis a triangular shape formed by _____ , _____ and _____ .

2. The anterior wall of axilla is formed by _____ , _____ , _____ and

   _____ .

3. The posterior wall of the axilla consists of _____ , _____ , _____ and

   _____ .

4. The structures passing through the clavipectoral fascia contain _____ , _____

   and _____ .

5. The axillary artery is divided into _____ segments by _____ as a mark.

6. The trilateral space transmits _____ ; the quadrilateral space transmits _____

   and _____ .

7. Axillary lymph nodes are arranged along the neurovascular bundle in the axilla and are

   divided into five groups, such as _____ , _____ , _____ , _____

   and _____ .

8. The scapular arterial network is located around the scapula and consists of branches of

   _____ , _____ and _____ .

9. Fractures of the surgical neck of the humerus can injure _____ and result in del-

   toid paralysis.

10. The shoulder sleeve is formed by the tendons of _____ , _____ , _____

    and _____ adhering with shoulder capsule.

IV. Answer the questions briefly

1. Please describe the boundaries of quadrangular space and contents passing through it.

2. Please describe the formation of anterior wall of axilla.

3. Please describe the constituents of shoulder cuff.

4. Please describe the divisions and branches of axillary artery.

5. Please describe the axillary lymph nodes.

V. Answer the questions in detail

1. Please describe the formation of the axilla.

2. Please describe the contents of the axilla.

Section 3   The Arm

Outline and Objectives

I . Grasp

1. The names, origin, insertion, nerve supplying and actions of the muscles (biceps brachii, coracobrachialis, brachialis) of the anterior group of arm.
2. The origin, insertion, nerve supplying and actions of the triceps brachii.
3. The formation and contents of the humeromuscular tunnel.
4. The contents of the medial bicipital groove.
5. The branches of brachial artery in arm.

II . Comprehend

1. The characteristics of the skin and superficial fascia.
2. The general situation and distribution of the cutaneous nerves in arm.
3. The contents of the lateral bicipital groove.
4. The structures of the cross-section through the middle of the arm.

Exercises

I . Single choice (Choose the best answer among the following four answers, and write the corresponding letter in the bracket)

1. Which description of the course of radial nerve in the arm is **wrong**? (   )

    A. It runs in front of the brachial artery in the upper arm.

    B. It runs along the sulcus for radial nerve with deep brachial artery.

    C. It passes through the humeromuscular tunnel to the posterior region of arm.

    D. It lies in the groove for radial nerve in the middle part of the humerus.

2. Which structure passes through the medial bicipital groove as follows? (   )

    A. Brachial vessels and median nerve

    B. Brachial vessels, median nerve and basilic vein

    C. Brachial vessels, median nerve and radial nerve

    D. Brachial vessels, median nerve and cephalic vein

3. The nerve distributed in the skin of the lower medial side of arm is (   ).

    A. medial brachial cutaneous nerve

    B. intercostobrachial nerve

    C. medial cutaneous nerve of forearm

    D. lateral brachial cutaneous nerve

4. The nerve passing through the humeromuscular tunnel is (　　).
   A. ulnar nerve
   B. axillary nerve
   C. musculocutaneous nerve
   D. radial nerve
5. The artery passing through the humeromuscular tunnel is (　　).
   A. brachial artery
   B. ulnar artery
   C. deep brachial artery
   D. radial artery
6. Which one is easily injured because of fracture of the shaft of humerus? (　　)
   A. Musculocutaneous nerve
   B. Radial nerve
   C. Median nerve
   D. Axillary nerve
7. The structures of the anterior osteofascial compartment of arm do **not** include (　　).
   A. musculocutaneous nerve
   B. ulnar nerve
   C. axillary nerve
   D. median nerve
8. Musculocutaneous nerve is **not** distributed in (　　).
   A. biceps brachii
   B. brachialis
   C. coracobrachialis
   D. skin of lateral part of arm
9. The structure lying in posterior osteofascial compartment of arm is (　　).
   A. triceps brachii
   B. brachial artery
   C. axillary nerve
   D. radial artery
10. The structure emerging from lower part of the lateral bicipital groove is (　　).
    A. lateral cutaneous nerve of forearm
    B. cephalic vein
    C. superficial branch of radial nerve
    D. basilic vein

II. Double choices (Choose the two best answers among the following answers, and write the corresponding letters in the bracket)

1. About the descriptions of the humeromuscular tunnel, which of the following are correct?
   (　　)
   A. The brachial artery and radial nerve pass through it.

B. It is enclosed by biceps brachii and groove for radial nerve of humerus.

C. The deep brachial artery has no branches in it.

D. The radial nerve branches in it to innervate triceps brachii.

E. It is surrounded by triceps brachii and groove for radial nerve of humerus.

2. The branches of brachial artery in the arm do **not** include (　　).

A. ulnar artery

B. superior ulnar collateral artery

C. inferior ulnar collateral artery

D. radial artery

E. deep brachial artery

3. About the descriptions of deep brachial artery, which of the following are right? (　　)

A. It is companying with ulnar nerve.

B. It passes through the groove for radial nerve of humerus.

C. It is easily injured by fractures of surgical neck of humerus.

D. It supplies the posterior region of arm.

E. It comes from the third segment of the axillary artery.

4. The musculocutaneous nerve do **not** distribute in (　　).

A. biceps brachii

B. brachialis

C. coracobrachialis

D. deltoid

E. triceps brachii

5. The structures pass through the humeromuscular tunnel are (　　).

A. brachial artery

B. deep brachial artery

C. ulnar artery

D. radial nerve

E. musculocutaneous nerve

Ⅲ. Fill the blanks (Fill the most appropriate words and phrases in the blanks)

1. There are two sulci for nerves on the surface of humerus, behind the middle part of-shaft is _____.

2. When a fracture of shaft of humerus happens, _____ is easy to injure and result in the wrist drop.

3. The humeromuscular tunnel is surrounded by _____ and _____.

4. The cutaneous nerves distributed in the anterior area of arm are _____ , _____ , _____ and _____.

5. The contents of the medial bicipital groove are _____ , _____ , _____ , _____ and _____ etc.

6. There are _____ and _____ located in the humeromuscular tunnel.

7. The anterior osteofascial compartment of the arm contains _____ , _____ , _____ , _____ and upper part of _____ .

8. The branches of brachial artery in the arm are _____ , _____ , _____ and _____ .

9. The contents of the lateral bicipital groove are _____ and _____ .

10. The posterior osteofascial compartment of arm contains _____ , _____ and _____ .

IV. Answer the questions briefly

1. Please describe the humeromuscular tunnel and contents of it.
2. Please describe the neurovascular bundles of anterior part of arm.

V. Answer the questions in detail

Please describe the muscles of arm and nerve supplying of them.

Section 4   The Elbow

Outline and Objectives

I. Grasp

1. The formation (roof, floor and boundary) and contents of the cubital fossa.
4. The type and the clinic significance of the anastomosis of the superficial veins (cephalic, basilic and median cubital veins) of the anterior part of elbow.

II. Comprehend

1. The constitution and significance of the arterial network of the elbow joint.
2. The formation and contents of cubital tunnel (canal of ulnar nerve) as well as the significance.
3. The posterior cubital triangle and lateral cubital triangle.
4. The position, collection and drainage of the supratrochlear lymph nodes.

Exercises

I. Single choice (Choose the best answer among the following four answers, and write the corresponding letter in the bracket)

1. The inferiomedial boundary of the cubital fossa is (   ).
   A. brachialis
   B. pronator teres
   C. brachioradialis
   D. supinator

2. Which structure is **not** in the cubital fossa as follows? (　　)

    A. Median nerve

    B. Ulnar nerve

    C. Ulnar artery

    D. Radial artery

3. The structure lies in the center of cubital fossa is (　　).

    A. radial nerve

    B. median nerve

    C. brachial vessels

    D. tendon of biceps

4. The artery that does **not** form the arterial network of elbow is (　　).

    A. ulnar superior collateral artery

    B. ulnar inferior collateral artery

    C. posterior interosseous artery

    D. radial collateral artery

5. Which of the following descriptions of the cubital fossa is **incorrect**? (　　)

    A. The inferior lateral boundary is brachioradialis.

    B. The base is the line between the medial and lateral epicondyles of the humerus.

    C. The floor is aponeurosis of biceps brachii.

    D. The floor is brachialis and capsule of elbow.

6. Which one belongs to bony landmarks of posterior region of elbow? (　　)

    A. Olecranon of ulna

    B. Coracoid process of ulna

    C. Trochlear notch of ulna

    D. Head of radius

7. When dislocation of elbow or fracture of medial epicondyle of humerus occurs, the nerve that can be injured is (　　).

    A. radial nerve

    B. ulnar nerve

    C. lateral forearm cutaneous nerve

    D. median nerve

8. Superficial cubital lymph nodes are located (　　).

    A. above the medial epicondyle of the humerus

    B. below the medial epicondyle of the humerus

    C. superior to lateral epicondyle of humerus

    D. inferior to lateral epicondyle of humerus

9. The nerve emerging out of deep fascia of lateral side of elbow is (　　).

    A. radial nerve

    B. ulnar nerve

    C. lateral cutaneous nerve of forearm

    D. median nerve

10. Which one of the following structures does **not** form the elbow joint? (　　)

    A. Trochlea of humerus and trochlear notch of ulnar

    B. Head of radius and capitulum of humerus

    C. Radial notch of ulnar and head of radius

    D. Ulnar notch of radius and head of ulna

II. Double choices (Choose the two best answers among the following answers, and write the corresponding letters in the bracket)

1. About the following descriptions of the cubital fossa, which ones are correct? (　　)

    A. The lower lateral boundary is the pronator teres.

    B. The lower medial boundary is the brachioradialis.

    C. The tendon of biceps brachii is located in the center of the cubital fossa.

    D. The brachial vesselsare lateral to the tendon of biceps.

    E. The median nerve is medial to the tendon of biceps.

2. About the superficial structures in front of the elbow, which ones are correct? (　　)

    A. The cephalic vein and the lateral antebrachial cutaneous nerve run medially to the tendon of biceps brachii.

    B. The basilic vein and the medial antebrachial cutaneous nerve run laterally to the tendon of biceps brachii.

    C. The median cubital vein connects the cephalic vein with the basilic vein.

    D. The median antebrachial vein enters the cephalic and the basilic veins respectively sometimes.

    E. The superficial veins are fine, fixed and deeper using in clinic commonly.

3. The arteries that do **not** form the arterial network of elbow are (　　).

    A. superior ulnar collateral artery

    B. inferior ulnar collateral artery

    C. posterior interosseous artery

    D. interosseous recurrent artery

    E. anterior interosseous artery

4. The following structures are included in the cubital fossa, **except** (　　).

    A. brachial vessels

    B. deep brachial vessels

    C. ulnar nerve

    D. median nerve

    E. radial nerve

5. The bony landmarks in the posterior cubital area do **not** contain (   ).

    A. medial epicondyle of humerus.

    B. olecranon of ulna.

    C. lateral epicondyle of humerus.

    D. groove for ulnar nerve.

    E. trochlea of humerus.

Ⅲ. Fill the blanks (Fill the most appropriate words and phrases in the blanks)

1. The three important bony landmarks of the posterior region of elbow are _____ , _____ and _____ .

2. _____ vein with the lateral antebrachial cutaneous nerve lies on the lateral side of the elbow , and the _____ vein with the medial antebrachial cutaneous nerve lies on the medial side.

3. When the elbow is flexed to a right angle, _____ is formed by the lateral epicondyle, the head of radius and the olecranon.

4. The cubital fossa is located in front of _____ .

5. The lower medial boundary of cubital fossa is _____ , and the lower lateral boundary is _____ .

6. The base of the cubital fossa is composed of _____ and _____ .

7. The structure in the center of cubital fossa is _____ , media to it is _____ nerve and lateral one is _____ nerve.

8. Dislocation of elbow joint or fracture of medial epicondyle of humerus can injure _____ .

9. The brachial artery is divided into _____ artery and _____ artery.

10. The elbow joint is a compound joint, which includes _____ joint, _____ joint and _____ joint.

Ⅳ. Answer the questions briefly

1. Please describe the formation of arterial rete of elbow joint.

2. Please describe the posterior cubital triangle.

Ⅴ. Answer the questions in detail

Please describe the position, formation and contents of the cubital fossa.

Section 5   The Forearm

Outline and Objectives

Ⅰ. Grasp

1. The names, layers, position, nerve supplying and actions of the muscles of the anteri-

or group in the forearm.

2. The names, layers, position, nerve supplying and actions of the muscles of the posterior group in the forearm.

3. The position, course, branches and distribution of the blood vessels and the nerves in the anterior aspect of the forearm.

Ⅱ. Comprehend

1. The characteristics of the skin and superficial fascia.

2. The general situation and the distribution of the cutaneous nerves in the forearm.

3. The contents, course and distribution of the posterior interosseous neurovascular bundle.

4. The concept and significance of posterior flexor space of forearm.

Exercises

Ⅰ. Single choice (Choose the best answer among the following four answers, and write the corresponding letter in the bracket)

1. Which of the following muscles is innervated by posterior interosseous nerve? (　　)

    A. Flexor carpi radialis

    B. Brachioradialis

    C. Supination

    D. Extensor carpi radialis brevis

2. Which of the following muscles is innervated by anterior interosseous nerve? (　　)

    A. Pronation teres

    B. Pronator quadratus

    C. Supinator

    D. Flexor carpi radialis

3. The deep branch of radial nerve penetrates (　　).

    A. brachioradialis

    B. pronator teres

    C. supination

    D. quadrilateral space

4. About the descriptions of radial artery, which one is **wrong**? (　　)

    A. It is companion with superficial branch of radial nerve in middle forearm.

    B. It is accompanied by one same named vein.

    C. It is locatedon the deep side of brachioradialis.

    D. It can be touched at the bottom of anatomical snuffbox.

5. About the descriptions of the forearm, which one is right? (　　)

    A. Radial artery is located on the radial side of brachioradialis.

    B. The superficial branch of the radial nerve innervates flexor carpi radialis.

C. The anterior interosseous artery originates from the radial artery.

D. Deep branch of radial nerve penetrates supinator.

6. About the posterior muscles of forearm, which description is **wrong**? (   )

A. They lie in the posterior osteofascial compartment of forearm.

B. There are 10 muscles.

C. They are innervated by the radial nerve.

D. They are innervated by the radial and ulnar nerves.

7. About the anterior muscles of forearm, which description is **wrong**? (   )

A. They lie in the anterior osteofascial compartment of forearm.

B. They are innervated by median and ulnar nerves

C. They are innervated by the median, ulnar and radial nerves.

D. There are nine muscles.

8. Which one is between the superficial and deep muscles of back of forearm? (   )

A. Radial neurovascular bundle

B. Ulnar neurovascular bundle

C. Median neurovascular bundle

D. Posterior interosseous neurovascular bundle

9. The nerve supplying the skin of lateral side of forearm is (   ).

A. musculocutaneous nerve

B. ulnar nerve

C. median nerve

D. radial nerve

10. The descriptions of median nerve, which of the following is right? (   )

A. There are no braches in forearm.

B. It penetrates the supinator.

C. It penetrates the pronator teres.

D. It supplies flexor carpi ulnaris.

Ⅱ. **Double choices (Choose the two best answers among the following answers, and write the corresponding letters in the bracket)**

1. The nerves supplying of anterior muscles of forearm do **not** include? (   )

A. Radial nerve

B. Musculocutaneous nerve

C. Median nerve

D. Ulnar nerve

E. Axillary nerve

2. Which ones do **not** belong to contents of radial neurovascular bundle? (   )

A. Radial artery

B. Radial veins

C. Superficial branch of radial nerve

D. Posterior interosseous nerve

E. Posterior interosseous artery

3. Which ones belong to neurovascular bundles of anterior region of forearm? (   )

A. Radial neurovascular bundle

B. Ulnar neurovascular bundle

C. Median neurovascular bundle

D. Brachial vessels

E. Posterior interosseous neurovascular bundle

4. About the following descriptions of forearm, which ones are **wrong**? (   )

A. The common interosseous artery comes from ulnar artery.

B. The common interosseous artery comes from radial artery.

C. The supinator is supplied by posterior interosseous nerve.

D. The brachioradialis is supplied by median nerve.

E. The ulnar artery lies lateral to the flexor carpi ulnaris.

5. The muscles supplied by median nerve include (   ).

A. flexor carpi radialis

D. flexor carpi ulnaris

C. pronator teres

D. supinator

E. brachioradialis

Ⅲ. Fill the blanks (Fill the most appropriate words and phrases in the blanks)

1. The superficial veins of the forearm are _____ and _____, accompanied by _____ and _____ nerve respectively.

2. The muscles flexing wrist include _____, _____, _____, _____, _____ and _____.

3. The muscles extending wrist include _____, _____, _____, _____, _____ and _____.

4. The muscles of forearm rotating anteriorly are _____ and _____.

5. The muscles of forearm rotating posteriorly are _____ and _____.

6. The nerves in anterior osteofascial compartment of forearm include _____, _____ and _____.

7. The radial neurovascular bundle consists of _____, _____ and _____.

8. The anterior interosseous neurovascular bundle contains _____ and _____.

Ⅳ. Answer the questions briefly

1. Please describe the neurovascular bundles of forearm.

2. Please describe the nerve supplying of anterior group muscles of forearm.

V. Answer the questions in detail

1. Please describe the formation and contents of anterior osteofascial compartment of forearm.

2. Please describe the formation and contents of posterior osteofascial compartment of forearm.

Section 6   The Wrist and Hand

Outline and Objectives

I. Grasp

1. The formation of the carpal canal and the contents through it.

2. The characteristics of the stratification of the structures in the palm.

3. The formation and branches of the superficial and deep palmar arches.

4. The course and branches of median and ulnar nerves in the palm.

5. The structures of the palmar surface of the fingers.

II. Comprehend

1. The flexor retinaculum, carpal ulnar and carpal radial canals.

2. The muscles of the hand and the osteofascial compartments of the palm.

3. The fascial spaces of palm

4. The stratification of the dorsum of the hand.

5. The general situation and the distribution of the cutaneousnerves in the hand.

Exercises

I. Single choice (Choose the best answer among the following four answers, and write the corresponding letter in the bracket)

1. The flexor retinaculum does **not** attach to the (   ).

   A. pisiform

   B. hamate

   C. scaphoid

   D. trapezoid

2. The structure passing through carpal canal is the (   ).

   A. ulnar nerve

   B. tendon of flexor carpi radialis

   C. tendon of flexor pollicis longus

   D. radial nerve

3. The tendon of flexor carpi radialis and its sheath lies in (   ).

 A. ulnar carpal canal

 B. radial carpal canal

 C. carpal canal

 D. humeral muscle tube

4. About the anatomical snuffbox, which description is right? (   )

 A. The lateral boundary is tendon of extensor pollicis longus.

 B. The medial border is the tendon of extensor pollicis brevis.

 C. The distal boundary is styloid process of radius.

 D. The radial artery passes through it.

5. About the following description of superficial palmar arch, which one is right? (   )

 A. It is superficial to the palmar aponeurosis.

 B. It lies in midpalmar space.

 C. It lies in intermediate compartment of palm.

 D. It lies in lateral compartment of palm.

6. The nerve innervating the adductor pollicis is (   ).

 A. axillary nerve

 B. radial nerve

 C. median nerve

 D. ulnar nerve

7. The deep palmar arch is composed of (   ).

 A. the terminal branch of radial artery and the deep palmar branch of ulnar artery

 B. the terminal branch of the radial artery and the superficial palmar branch of the ulnar artery

 C. the superficial palmar branch of the radial artery and terminal branch of the ulnar artery

 D. the superficial palmar branch of the radial artery and deep branch of the ulnar artery

8. Which of the following structures does not passing through ulnar carpal canal? (   )

 A. Tendon of flexor carpi ulnaris

 B. Radial artery

 C. Ulnar nerve

 D. Ulnar vein

9. The nerve innervating the 1st and 2nd lumbrical muscles is (   ).

 A. radial nerve

 B. ulnar nerve

 C. median nerve

 D. recurrent branch of median nerve

10. The nerve innervating the 3rd and 4th lumbrical muscles is (   ).

 A. radial nerve

  B. ulnar nerve

  C. median nerve

  D. recurrent branch of median nerve

II. Double choices (Choose the two best answers among the following answers, and write the corresponding letters in the bracket)

  1. The osteofascial compartments of the palm do **not** include ( ).

    A. medial compartment

    B. lateral compartment

    C. intermediate compartment

    D. common flexor sheath

    E. tendinous sheath of flexor pollicis longus

  2. The fascial spaces of palm contain ( ).

    A. midpalmar space

    B. thenar space

    C. hypothenar space

    D. posterior adductor pollicis space

    E. posterior flexor space

  3. The nerves supplying thenar muscles are ( ).

    A. radial nerve

    B. median nerve

    C. ulnar nerve

    D. anterior interosseous nerve

    E. posterior interosseous nerve

  4. The following structures lie superficial to carpal canal are ( ).

    A. tendon of flexor digitorum

    B. median nerve

    C. ulnar nerve

    D. palmar aponeurosis

    E. tendon of flexor pollicis longus

  5. The following structures formed by flexor retinaculum are ( ).

    A. posterior flexor space of forearm

    B. ulnar carpal canal

    C. radial carpal canal

    D. carpal canal

    E. common flexor sheath

III. Fill the blanks (Fill the most appropriate words and phrases in the blanks)

  1. The flexor retinaculum is attached to _____ , _____ and _____ medially, and _____ laterally.

2. The radial carpal canal transmits _____ .

3. The ulnar carpal canal contains _____ , _____ and _____ .

4. The tendons of carpal extensor and tendinous sheath passing within the osteofibrous canals arranged from lateral to medial are _____ , _____ , _____ , _____ and _____ .

5. The two fascial spaces in the palm are _____ and _____ .

IV. Answer the questions briefly

1. Please describe the formation and contents of carpal canal.

2. Please describe the formation of the anatomical snuffbox.

3. Please describe the nerve distribution of skin on the hand.

V. Answer the questions in detail

1. Please describe the layers of palm.

2. Please describe the osteofascial compartments of the palm.

Chapter 4　The Lower Limb

Section 1　Introduction

Outline and Objectives

I. Grasp

1. The start-stop, courses, tributaries and clinical notes of the great saphenous vein, and small saphenous vein.
2. The situation, divided groups and collecting area of the superficial inguinal lymph nodes.
3. The principal features of the hip bone, femur, tibia and fibula.
4. The composition, structural features and movement of the hip joint, knee joint and ankle joint.
5. The surface landmarks of the lower limb.

II. Comprehend

1. The boundary and partition of the lower limb.
2. The stratification of the structure of the human body.
3. The distribution of the cutaneous nerves in the lower limb.
4. The structures met in dissection.
5. The names and arrangement of the bones of the lower limb.

Exercises

I. Single choice (Choose the best answer among the following four answers, and write the corresponding letter in the bracket)

1. Which of the following is the thickest nerve in the body? (　　)
   A. The inferior gluteal nerve
   B. The superior gluteal nerve
   C. The sciatic nerve
   D. The femoral nerve
2. Which of the following is the surface landmarks of the foot? (　　)
   A. The neck of the fibula

B. The lateral malleolus

C. The tendon of the biceps femoris

D. The shaft of the tibia

3. Which of the following belongs to the foot region? (   )

A. The anterior region

B. The posterior region

C. The medial region

D. The dorsum

Ⅱ. **Double choices (Choose the two best answers among the following answers, and write the corresponding letters in the bracket)**

1. Which are the surface landmarks of the knee? (   )

A. The tendon of the biceps femoris

B. The neck of the fibula

C. The tendon of semitendinosus

D. The greater trochanter

E. The inguinal ligament

2. Which are the surface landmarks of the leg? (   )

A. The tendon of the biceps femoris

B. The neck of the fibula

C. The tendo calcaneus

D. The medial malleolus

E. The shaft of the tibia

3. Which of the following parts belong to the lower limb? (   )

A. The elbow

B. The gluteal region

C. The leg

D. The shoulder

E. The arm

Ⅲ. **Fill the blanks (Fill the most appropriate words and phrases in the blanks)**

1. The lower limb can be divided into following parts:_____ ,_____ ,_____ and _____ .

2. The pulsation of the foot is palpable from the _____ midpoint between the malleoli and the proximal end of the first intermetatarsal space.

3. Surface projection of the begins 2. 5cm distal to the medial _____ , side of the fibular head and ends midpoint between the malleoli.

4. The thickest nerve in the body is _____ .

Ⅳ. Answer the questions briefly

1. The boundaries of the lower limb.

2. The divisions of the lower limb.

3. The surface landmarks of the gluteal region and thigh.

4. The surface landmarks of the foot.

5. The projections of the inferior gluteal artery, vein, and nerve.

Section 2   The Gluteal Region

Outline and Objectives

Ⅰ. Grasp

1. The layers and names of the gluteal muscles, such as gluteus maximus, gluteus medius, gluteus minimus, piriformis, tensor fasciae latae, obturator internus and quadratus femoris.

2. The origin, insertion, action and nerve supply of gluteus maximus and piriformis.

3. The structures passing through the suprapiriform foramen.

4. The structures passing through the infrapiriform foramen.

5. The constitution of the lesser sciatic foramen and the vessels and nerves passing through the foramen.

6. The origin, course and distribution of the sciatic nerve.

7. The structures exit the greater sciatic foramen.

8. The ligaments and foramina of the gluteal region.

9. The composition, structural features and movement of the hip joint.

Ⅱ. Comprehend

1. The name, position and nerve supply of muscles of the gluteal region.

2. The boundary and surface anatomy of the gluteal region.

3. The characteristics of the skin and the superficial fascia.

4. The surface projection of the sciatic nerve.

5. The formation and the practical significance of the arterial rete around the hip joint.

Exercises

Ⅰ. Single choice (Choose the best answer among the following four answers, and write the corresponding letter in the bracket)

1. Which of the following statements concerning the lesser sciatic foramen is correct?
   (   )

   A. All arteries and nerves of lower limb leave the pelvis through this foramen.

B. The obturator nerve enters the adductor compartment via the lesser sciatic foramen.

C. It is the passageway for structures entering or leaving the perineum.

D. It is the passageway for structures entering or leaving the pelvis.

2. All of the following structures pass through the greater sciatic foramen **except** (　　).

A. piriformis

B. femoral nerve

C. sciatic nerve

D. superior gluteal vessels

3. Which of the following statements concerning the gluteus medius and minimus is **wrong**? (　　)

A. They all have the same nerve supply.

B. They have the same actions.

C. They are supplied by the same blood vessels.

D. They adduct the thigh and rotate it medially.

4. Which of the following statements concerning the sciatic nerve is **wrong**? (　　)

A. It is the largest nerve in the body.

B. It is divided into two branches.

C. It supplies all muscles of leg and foot.

D. It is divided into three branches.

5. Which of the following structures passes through the greater sciatic foramen? (　　)

A. The piriformis

B. The femoral nerve

C. The obturator nerve

D. The greater saphenous vein

6. Which of the following cutaneous nerves to supply the lower lateral part of the gluteal region? (　　)

A. The subcostal nerve

B. The lateral cutaneous branch of iliohypogastric nerve

C. The posterior branch of lateral femoral cutaneous nerve

D. The inferior cluneal nerves

7. Which of the following cutaneous nerves curve around the lower border of the gluteus maximus to supply the lower part of the gluteal region? (　　)

A. The inferior cluneal nerves

B. The superior cluneal nerves

C. The posterior branch of lateral femoral cutaneous nerve

D. The medial cluneal nerves

8. Which of the following cutaneous nerves to supply the medial part ofthe gluteal region? (　　)

A.The subcostal nerve

B.The medial cluneal nerves

C.The posterior branch of lateral femoral cutaneous nerve

D.The lateral cutaneous branch of iliohypogastric nerve

9. Which of following structures passes through the infrapiriform foramen? (　　)

A. The superior gluteal artery

B. The femoral nerve

C. The sciatic nerve

D. The superior gluteal nerve

10. Which of following structures passes through the suprapiriform foramen? (　　)

A. The superior gluteal artery

B. The femoral nerve

C. The pudendal nerve

D. The inferior gluteal artery

Ⅱ. Double choices (Choose the two best answers among the following answers, and write the corresponding letters in bracket)

1. Which of the following muscles are supplied by the deep branches of superior gluteal artery? (　　)

A. The gluteus medius

B. The piriformis

C. The gluteus minimus

D. The obturator internus

E. The obturator externus

2. Which of the following muscles belong to the gluteal region? (　　)

A. The quadriceps femoris

B. The gluteus maximus

C. The adductor magnus

D. The gracilis

E. The gluteus minimus

3. Which of the following cutaneous nerves to supply the upper lateral part of the gluteal region? (　　)

A. The posterior branch of lateral femoral cutaneous nerve

B. The subcostal nerve

C. The inferior cluneal nerves

D. The lateral cutaneous branch of iliohypogastric nerve

E. The superior cluneal nerves

4. Which of the following structures pass through the infrapiriform foramen? （　　）
   A. The sciatic nerve
   B. The femoral nerve
   C. The superior gluteal artery
   D. The inferior gluteal artery
   E. The superior gluteal nerve
5. Which of the following structures pass through the suprapiriform foramen? （　　）
   A. The pudendal nerve
   B. The femoral nerve
   C. The superior gluteal artery
   D. The inferior gluteal artery
   E. The superior gluteal nerve
6. Which of the following muscles are the superficial layer of the gluteal region? （　　）
   A. The gluteus maximus
   B. The tensor fasciae latae
   C. The tendon of obturator internus
   D. The quadratus femoris
   E. The piriformis
7. Which of the following arteries are the superficial blood vessels of the gluteal region?
   （　　）
   A. The inferior gluteal artery
   B. The lateral sacral artery
   C. The 4th lumbar artery
   D. The musculocutaneous artery
   E. The cutaneous artery

Ⅲ. Fill the blanks （Fill the most appropriate words and phrases in the blanks）

1. _____ supplies the lower lateral part of the gluteal region.
2. The inferior cluneal nerve to supply the _____ .
3. _____ is a very large muscle and is the most superficial in the gluteal region.
4. _____ arises from the ventral surface of the sacrum and runs laterally through _____ to converge on the medial border of the greater trochanter.
5. The superior gluteal artery arises from the posterior aspect of the _____ .

Ⅳ. Answer the questions briefly

1. The superficial blood and lymph vessels of the gluteal region.
2. The cutaneous nerves of the gluteal region.

Ⅴ. Answer the questions in detail

1. Describe the course, distribution and relationship of the sciatic nerve.
2. Describe the structures pass through the suprapiriform foramen.
3. Describe the structures pass through the infrapiriform foramen.

Section 3　The Thigh

Outline and Objectives

Ⅰ. Grasp

1. The names, positional relation, start-stop, supplied nerves and actions of the muscles of the anterior and medial groups in the thigh.
2. The names, position, start-stop and supplied nerves of the muscles of the posterior group in the thigh.
3. The beginnings, course, tributaries and endings of great saphenous vein.
4. The position and area drainage of the deep inguinal lymph nodes.
5. The boundaries and contents of the femoral triangle.
6. The composition and contents of the femoral sheath.
7. The boundaries and contents of the femoral ring.
8. The beginning, ending and branches of the femoral artery.
9. The origin, branches and distribution of the femoral nerve.
10. The position and area drainage of the superficial inguinal lymph nodes.
11. The origin, insertion, action and nerve supply of sartorius and quadriceps femoris.
12. The position, formation and the passing structures of the adductor canal.

Ⅱ. Comprehend

1. The boundary and surface anatomy of the anterior and medial region of the thigh.
2. The characteristics of the skin and the superficial fascia.
3. The structures formed by the deep fascia of the thigh (saphenous hiatus and iliotibial tract).
4. The distributions of the superficial blood vessels and the cutaneous nerves.
5. The contents of anterior, medial and posterior fascial compartment of the thigh.
6. The situation, divided groups and drainage relation of the superficial lymph nodes.
7. The beginning, branches and distribution of the obturator nerve.
8. The beginning, branches and distribution of the obturator artery.
9. The anatomy of the cross-section through the middle of the thigh.

Exercises

Ⅰ. Single choice (Choose the best answer among the following four answers, and write the corresponding letter in the bracket)

1. Which of the following structures covers the saphenous hiatus? (　　)
    A. Cribriform fascia

B. Iliotibial tract

C. Lateral intermuscular septum

D. Medial intermuscular septum

2. Which of the following structures passes through the saphenous hiatus? (   )

A. The femoral artery

B. The great saphenous vein

C. The femoral nerve

D. The obturator nerve

3. Which of the following is the longest branch of the femoral nerve? (   )

A. The anterior cutaneous branches of the femoral nerve

B. The lateral femoral cutaneous nerve

C. The ilioinguinal nerve

D. The saphenous nerve

4. Which of the following is the deep fascia of the thigh? (   )

A. Scarpa's fascia

B. Colles' fascia

C. Plantar fascia

D. Fascia lata

5. About the iliopsoas, which of the following statements is correct? (   )

A. It is a flat quadrangular muscle.

B. It is the chief flexor of the thigh.

C. It is enclosed between two layers of fascia lata.

D. It inserts into the iliotibial tract.

6. About the sartorius, which of the following statements is **wrong**? (   )

A. It is the longest muscle in the body.

B. It is the chief flexor of the thigh.

C. It acts across two joints.

D. It extends the hip.

7. About the gracilis, which of the following statements is correct? (   )

A. It passes through the lesser sciatic foramen.

B. It crosses the knee joint.

C. It lies deep to the pectineus and adductor longus.

D. It is located in the anterior compartment of the thigh.

8. Which structure is **not** in the adductor canal? (   )

A. Femoral artery

B. Femoral vein

C. Femoral nerve

D. Saphenous nerve

9. In the femoral triangle, what is the arrangement of the femoral artery, femoral vein and femoral nerve? (   )

   A. Lateral is femoral nerve, middle is femoral vein and medial is femoral artery.

   B. Lateral is femoral artery, middle is femoral vein and medial is femoral nerve.

   C. Lateral is femoral nerve, middle is femoral artery and medial is femoral vein.

   D. Lateral is femoral vein, middle is femoral nerve and medial is femoral artery.

10. About the lacuna vasorum, which of the following statements is **wrong**? (   )

   A. Anterior border is the inguinal ligament.

   B. Posterior border is the pectineal ligament.

   C. Medial border is lacunar ligament.

   D. Medial border is iliopectineal arch.

11. Which structure may be found in the lacuna musculorum? (   )

   A. Femoral nerve

   B. Saphenous nerve

   C. Great saphenous vein

   D. Femoral artery

12. Which structure is **not** in the femoral sheath? (   )

   A. Femoral artery

   B. Femoral vein

   C. Femoral nerve

   D. Femoral canal

13. Which one does **not** belong to tributaries of great saphenous vein? (   )

   A. Superficial epigastric vein

   B. Internal pudendal vein

   C. Superficial lateral femoral vein

   D. Superficial medial femoral vein

14. About the femoral artery, which of the following statements is correct? (   )

   A. It enters the femoral canal.

   B. It enters the adductor canal.

   C. It gives rise to the inferior epigastric artery.

   D. It passes through the obturator canal.

15. About the deep artery of the thigh, which of the following statements is correct? (   )

   A. It is the largest branch of the femoral artery.

   B. It passes through the adductor canal.

   C. It gives rise to the deep circumflex iliac branch.

   D. It passes through the obturator foramen.

16. About the adductor canal, which of the following statements is **wrong**? (   )

   A. It is approximately 15 cm long.

   B. It extends from the apex of the femoral triangle to the adductor hiatus.

     C. It contains the saphenous nerve.

     D. It's bounded posteriorly by the sartorius.

17. About the adductor tendinous opening, which of the following statements is correct? (　　)

     A. It transmits the femoral nerve, artery and vein.

     B. The opening is located just inferior to the adductor tubercle of the femur.

     C. It extends from the adductor canal in the thigh to the popliteal fossa.

     D. The great saphenous vein passes through it.

18. Which nerve does **not** arise from the lumbar plexus? (　　)

     A. Femoral nerve

     B. Obturator nerve

     C. Sciatic nerve

     D. Lateral femoral cutaneous nerve

19. Which of the following is the superior border of the femoral triangle? (　　)

     A. Adductor longus

     B. Inguinal ligament

     C. Fascia lata

     D. Iliopsoas

20. Which of the following is the anterior border of the adductor canal? (　　)

     A. Adductors longus

     B. Adductor lamina

     C. Adductors magnus

     D. Vastus medialis

II. Double choices (Choose the two best answers among the following answers, and write the corresponding letters in the bracket)

1. Which are the tributaries of the great saphenous vein? (　　)

     A. The superficial epigastric vein

     B. The external pudendal vein

     C. The femoral vein

     D. The inferior gluteal vein

     E. The internal pudendal vein

2. Which of the following are the contents of the lacuna musculorum? (　　)

     A. The femoral artery

     B. The femoral nerve

     C. The lateral femoral cutaneous nerve

     D. The femoral vein

     E. The femoral canal

3. Which of the following are the contents of the lacuna vasorum? (　　)

     A. The femoral vein

    B. The lateral femoral cutaneous nerve

    C. The iliopsoas

    D. The femoral artery

    E. The femoral nerve

4. About the quadriceps femoris, which of the following statements are **wrong**? (   )

    A. Collectively constitutes the largest and most powerful muscle group in the body.

    B. It is the great extensor of the thigh.

    C. It inserts onto the tibia.

    D. It forms the main bulk of the anterior thigh muscles.

    E. It just acts on the hip joint.

5. About the adductor magnus, which of the following statements are **wrong**? (   )

    A. It is the largest muscle in the adductor group.

    B. It is located in the posterior compartment of the thigh.

    C. It is located in the medial compartment of the thigh.

    D. It is supplied by sciatic nerve.

    E. Its main action is to adduct the thigh.

6. About the femoral triangle, which of the following statements are **wrong**? (   )

    A. Its superior border is the inguinal ligament.

    B. Its lateral border is the sartorius.

    C. Its medial border is the adductor magnus.

    D. The saphenous nerve passes through the femoral triangle.

    E. The sciatic nerve passes through the femoral triangle.

7. About the femoral sheath, which of the following statements are **wrong**? (   )

    A. It extends 3 to 4 cm inferior the inguinal ligament.

    B. It is formed by an inferior prolongation of transverse and iliopsoas fascia.

    C. The femoral artery lies the middle compartment.

    D. It contains the femoral nerve.

    E. The medial compartment is the femoral canal.

8. About the femoral canal, which of the following statements are **wrong**? (   )

    A. It is the medial compartment of the femoral sheath.

    B. It is the lateral compartment of the femoral sheath.

    C. It contains loose connective tissue, fat and lymphatic vessels.

    D. It contains the femoral nerve.

    E. It extends distally to the level of the proximal edge of the saphenous opening.

9. About the femoral ring, which of the following statements are **wrong**? (   )

    A. The lacunar ligament forms its medial boundary.

    B. The inguinal ligament forms its anterior boundary.

    C. The femoral vein forms its lateral boundary.

    D. The femoral artery forms its lateral boundary.

    E. It lies posterior to the pectineus.

10. Which of the following are the branches of the deep femoral artery? (   )

    A. The lateral femoral circumflex artery

    B. The obturator artery

    C. The superficial epigastric artery

    D. The medial femoral circumflex artery

    E. The external pudendal artery

Ⅲ. Fill the blanks（Fill the most appropriate words and phrases in the blanks）

1. In front of upper part of the thigh, the superficial fascia consists of the superficial _____ and the deep _____ .

2. The femoral artery gives off three small arteries when it enters the femoral triangle: __ _____ artery, _____ artery and _____ arteries.

3. The longest branch of the femoral nerve is _____ .

4. A thickened band of deep fascia on the lateral side of the thigh and is known as the __ _____ .

5. The anterior osteofascial compartment of the thigh includes two muscles, _____ and _____ .

6. _____ occupies the lateral compartment of the femoral sheath. _____ lies the middle compartment.

7. The floor of the femoral triangle is formed by _____ , _____ and _____ , it's from medial to the lateral side.

8. _____ is the medial compartment of the femoral sheath.

9. The superior opening of the femoral canal is called the _____ .

10. The branches of the deep femoral artery are _____ , _____ and _____ .

11. The femoral nerve arises from the in the abdomen _____ .

12. The obturator artery arises from the internal iliac artery in the lesser pelvis, passes through the _____ and divides into anterior and poster branches.

13. The muscles of the back of the thigh are the _____ on the lateral side, the superficial _____ and deep _____ on the medial side.

14. In the lower third of the thigh, the sciatic nerve divides into _____ and _____ .

15. _____ is the largest and thickest walled superficial vein of the lower limb.

Ⅳ. Answer the questions briefly

1. The boundaries and contents of the lacuna musculorum.

2. The contents of the posterior osteofascial compartment of the thigh.

3. The boundaries and contents of the lacuna vasorum.

4. The composition and contents of the femoral sheath.

5. The boundaries and contents of the adduct canal.

V. Answer the questions in detail

1. Describe the boundaries and contents of the femoral triangle.

2. Describe the beginnings, course, endings and the tributaries of greater saphenous vein.

Section 4　The Knee

Outline and Objectives

I. Grasp

1. The boundaries of the popliteal fossa.

2. The contents of the popliteal fossa.

3. The branches and distribution of the popliteal artery.

4. The composition, structural features and movement of the knee joint.

II. Comprehend

1. The formation and the practical significance of the arterial rete around the knee joint.

2. The popliteal vein and its tributaries.

3. The popliteal lymph nodes.

Exercises

I. Single choice (Choose the best answer among the following four answers, and write the corresponding letter in the bracket)

1. The upper lateral boundary of the popliteal fossa is formed by the (　　).

A. biceps femoris

B. semitendinosus

C. semimembranosus

D. gastrocnemius

2. Which one belongs to intracapsular ligament? (　　)

A. The cruciate ligament

B. The iliofemoral ligament

C. The patellar ligament

D. The annular ligament of radius

3. The most complex joint in the body is (　　).

A. hip joint

B. shoulder joint

C. elbow joint

D. knee joint

4. The small saphenous vein empties into (　　).

   A. femoral vein

   B. popliteal vein

   C. superficial epigastric vein

   D. superficial iliac circumflex vein

5. About the popliteal fossa, which of the following is **wrong**? (　　)

   A. The semimembranosus forms the superomedial border.

   B. It contains both the tibial and common peroneal nerves.

   C. The lateral and medial heads of the gastrocnemius form the inferolateral and inferomedial borders.

   D. It contains the great saphenous vein.

6. The roof of the popliteal fossa is formed by the (　　).

   A. popliteal surface of femur

   B. semitendinosus

   C. semimembranosus

   D. popliteal fascia

7. The lateral sural nerve arise from (　　).

   A. femoral nerve

   B. common peroneal nerve

   C. obturator nerve

   D. tibial nerve

8. The medial sural nerve arise from (　　).

   A. femoral nerve

   B. superficial peroneal nerve

   C. deep peroneal nerve

   D. tibial nerve

9. All of the following structures of the knee are intra-articular **except** (　　).

   A. anterior cruciate ligament

   B. medial meniscus

   C. patellar ligament

   D. posterior cruciate ligament

10. Which of the following muscles is the most important muscle in stabilizing the knee?

   (　　)

   A. Biceps femoris

   B. Adductor magnus

   C. Quadriceps femoris

   D. Piriformis

II. Double choices (Choose the two best answers among the following answers, and write the corresponding letters in the bracket)

1. The upper medial boundary of the popliteal fossa is formed by the (   ).

   A. biceps femoris

   B. semitendinosus

   C. semimembranosus

   D. gastrocnemius

   E. popliteal fascia

2. Which of the following are the contents of the popliteal fossa? (   )

   A. Femoral vein

   B. Popliteal vessels

   C. Iliopsoas

   D. Femoral artery

   E. Small saphenous vein

3. Which of the following are the branches of common peroneal nerve? (   )

   A. Medial sural cutaneous nerve

   B. Superficial peroneal nerve

   C. Deep peroneal nerve

   D. Femoral nerve

   E. Saphenous nerve

4. Which of the following are the branches of the popliteal artery? (   )

   A. Anterior tibial artery

   B. Posterior tibial artery

   C. Superficial epigastric artery

   D. Femoral artery

   E. Superficial iliac circumflexartery

III. Fill the blanks (Fill the most appropriate words and phrases in the blanks)

1. The menisci are divided into the _____ and _____.

2. The cruciate ligament is divided into the _____ and _____.

3. The blood supply of the knee joint comes from the genicular branches of the _____.

4. The deep fascia of the popliteal fossa is called the _____.

IV. Answer the questions briefly

1. The course of popliteal vein.

2. The branches of common peroneal nerve in the popliteal fossa.

3. The branches of tibial nerve in the popliteal fossa.

4. The course, endings and the branches of popliteal artery.

V. Answer the questions in detail

Describe the boundaries and contents of the popliteal fossa.

Section 5   The Leg

Outline and Objectives

I. Grasp

1. The names, arrangement, start-stop, supplied nerves and actions of the muscles of the anterior and lateral groups in the leg.
2. The layers, names, start-stop, supplied nerves and actions of the posterior group in the leg.
3. The beginnings, course and endings of small saphenous vein.
4. The beginning, ending and branches of the anterior tibial artery.
5. The course, distribution and the clinical significance of the superficial peroneal verve.
6. The distributions of the deep peroneal nerves.
7. The origin, insertion, action and nerve supply of tibialis anterior, gastrocnemius and soleus and tibialis posterior.
8. The beginning, ending and branches of the posterior tibial artery.
9. The distributions of the tibial nerve.
10. The position, constitution and the passing structures of the malleolar canal.

II. Comprehend

1. The anatomy of the cross-section through the middle of the leg.
2. The contents of anterior and lateral fascial compartment of the leg.
3. The contents of posterior fascial compartment of the leg.

Exercises

I. Single choice (Choose the best answer among the following four answers, and write the corresponding letter in the bracket)

1. The great saphenous vein lies (   ).
   A. on the lateral side of the leg
   B. anterior to the medial malleolus
   C. posterior to the lateral malleolus
   D. on the back of the leg
2. The nerve accompanying with the great saphenous vein is (   ).
   A. femoral nerve
   B. superficial peroneal nerve

    C. tibial nerve

    D. saphenous nerve

3. About the small saphenous vein, which of the statements is **wrong**? (   )

    A. It arises from the dorsal venous arch of the foot.

    B. It lies behind the lateral malleolus.

    C. It accompanies with the saphenous nerve.

    D. It drains into the popliteal vein.

4. Which nerve innervates the skin of the medial side of foot? (   )

    A. Sural nerve

    B. Saphenous nerve

    C. Superficial peroneal nerve

    D. Deep peroneal nerve

5. Which nerve innervates the skin of the lower part of anterolateral surface of the leg?

    (   )

    A. Tibial nerve

    B. Common peroneal nerve

    C. Superficial peroneal nerve

    D. Deep peroneal nerve

6. Which one does **not** lie in the anterior osteofascial compartment of leg? (   )

    A. Tibialis anterior

    B. Flexor hallucis longus

    C. Extensor digitorum longus

    D. Anterior tibial artery

7. The muscle which lies in the posterior osteofascial compartment of leg is (   ).

    A. tibialis anterior

    B. gastrocnemius

    C. extensor digitorum longus

    D. extensor hallucis longus

8. Which one does **not** lie in the lateral osteofascial compartment of leg? (   )

    A. Peroneus longus

    B. Peroneus brevis

    C. Superficial peroneal nerve

    D. Deep peroneal nerve

9. The artery which lies in the anterior osteofascial compartment of leg is (   ).

    A. anterior tibial artery

    B. posterior tibial artery

    C. peroneal artery

    D. popliteal artery

10. The nerve innervating the muscles of anterior osteofascial compartment of leg is (   ).

   A. tibial nerve

   B. common peroneal nerve

   C. superficial peroneal nerve

   D. deep peroneal nerve

11. The nerve innervating the muscles of posterior osteofascial compartment of leg is (   ).

   A. tibial nerve

   B. common peroneal nerve

   C. superficial peroneal nerve

   D. deep peroneal nerve

12. The nerve innervating the muscles of lateral osteofascial compartment of leg is (   ).

   A. tibial nerve

   B. common peroneal nerve

   C. superficial peroneal nerve

   D. deep peroneal nerve

13. The following structures lie posterior to the lateral malleolus **except** (   ).

   A. small saphenous vein

   B. great saphenous vein

   C. peroneus longus

   D. peroneus brevis

14. Which one is **not** the branch of the superficial peroneal nerve? (   )

   A. Medial sural cutaneous nerve

   B. Lateral sural cutaneous nerve

   C. Medial dorsal cutaneous nerve

   D. Intermediate dorsal cutaneous nerve

15. Which of the following accompanies with the small saphenous vein? (   )

   A. Sural nerve

   B. Superficial peroneal nerve

   C. Deep peroneal nerve

   D. Tibial nerve

16. About the anterior tibial artery, which one is **wrong**? (   )

   A. It arises from the popliteal artery.

   B. It runs through the lateral osteofascial compartment of leg.

   C. In front of the ankle joint, it becomes the dorsal artery of foot.

   D. It supplies the muscles of anterior osteofascial compartment of leg.

17. Fracture of neck of fibula, which nerve is easily to be damaged? (   )

   A. Common peroneal nerve

   B. Superficial peroneal nerve

   C. Deep peroneal nerve

   D. Tibial nerve

18. The tendo calcaneus is formed by the tendons of gastrocnemius and (   ).

    A. popliteus

    B. flexor digitorum longus

    C. flexor hallucis longus

    D. soleus

19. The following muscles can plantar flex the foot **except** (   ).

    A. popliteus

    B. flexor digitorum longus

    C. flexor hallucis longus

    D. tibialis posterior

20. Which of the following is **not** the branch of posterior tibial artery? (   )

    A. Dorsal artery of foot

    B. Peroneal artery

    C. Medial plantar artery

    D. Lateral plantar artery

Ⅱ. **Double choices (Choose the two best answers among the following answers, and write the corresponding letters in the bracket)**

1. The structures running through the medial side of leg are(   ).

    A. great saphenous vein

    B. small saphenous vein

    C. saphenous nerve

    D. sural nerve

    E. superficial peroneal nerve

2. The muscles lying in the lateral osteofascial compartment of leg are (   ).

    A. peroneus longus

    B. peroneus brevis

    C. flexor digitorum longus

    D. flexor hallucis longus

    E. tibialis posterior

3. Which muscles are innervated by the tibial nerve? (   )

    A. Peroneus longus

    B. Tibialis anterior

    C. Flexor digitorum longus

    D. Flexor hallucis longus

    E. Peroneus brevis

4. The blood vessels and nerves in the anterior osteofascial compartment of leg are (   ).

    A. tibial nerve

    B. superficial peroneal nerve

　　C. deep peroneal nerve

　　D. anterior tibial vessels

　　E. posterior tibial vessels

　5. Sural nerve is formed by the union of (　　).

　　A. medial sural cutaneous nerve

　　B. lateral sural cutaneous nerve

　　C. medial dorsal cutaneous nerve

　　D. intermediate dorsal cutaneous nerve

　　E. saphenous nerve

Ⅲ. Fill the blanks (Fill the most appropriate words and phrases in the blanks)

　1. The great saphenous vein arises from the _____, and ascends in the medial side of leg accompanying with the _____.

　2. The muscles in the lateral osteofascial compartment of leg are _____ and _____; they are innervated by _____.

　3. The muscles in the anterior osteofascial compartment of leg are _____, _____ and _____; they are innervated by _____.

　4. The superficial vein in the posterior region of leg is _____, and its accompanying nerve is _____.

　5. The tendo calcaneus is formed by the tendons of _____ and _____.

　6. The skin of medial side of leg is innervated by _____, and it is a cutaneous branch of _____.

　7. There are two layers muscles in posterior osteofascial compartment of leg, the superficial layer contains _____, _____ and _____, deep layer contains _____, _____, _____ and _____.

　8. The cutaneous nerves in the posterior region of leg are _____, _____ and _____.

Ⅳ. Answer the questions briefly

　1. Briefly describe the contents of anterior osteofascial compartment of leg.

　2. Briefly describe the contents of lateral osteofascial compartment of leg.

　3. Briefly describe the superficial veins and cutaneous nerves of leg.

Ⅴ. Answer the questions in detail

　Describe the layers and contents of posterior osteofascial compartment of leg.

Section 6   The Ankle and Foot

Outline and Objectives

Ⅰ. Grasp

1. The position and the surface projection of the dorsal artery of the foot.
2. The composition, structural features and movement of the ankle joint.
3. The beginning, ending and branches of the dorsalis pedis artery.

Ⅱ. Comprehend

1. The superficial structures of the dorsum of the foot.
2. The positional relation of the medial and lateral plantar blood vessels and nerves.
3. The stratification of the muscles of the sole of the foot.
4. The composition of the arches of foot.
5. The muscles of the dorsum of the foot.

Exercises

Ⅰ. Single choice (Choose the best answer among the following four answers, and write the corresponding letter in the bracket)

1. The dorsal artery of foot is the continuation of (   ).
   A. peroneal artery
   B. anterior tibial artery
   C. posterior tibial artery
   D. popliteal artery
2. The intermediate dorsal cutaneous nerve is the branch of (   ).
   A. tibial nerve
   B. common peroneal nerve
   C. superficial peroneal nerve
   D. deep peroneal nerve
3. The skin of medial side of foot is innervated by (   ).
   A. sural nerve
   B. superficial peroneal nerve
   C. deep peroneal nerve
   D. saphenous nerve
4. The skin of lateral side of foot is innervated by (   ).
   A. sural nerve
   B. superficial peroneal nerve

C. deep peroneal nerve

D. saphenous nerve

5. The inferior extensor retinaculum holds the tendons of the following muscles **except** (   ).

A. tibialis anterior

B. tibialis posterior

C. extensor digitorum longus

D. extensor hallucis longus

6. The peroneal retinacula hold the tendon of (   ).

A. tibialis anterior

B. flexor digitorum longus

C. extensor digitorum longus

D. peroneus longus

7. The dorsal venous arch drains laterally into (   ).

A. anterior tibial vein

B. great saphenous vein

C. small saphenous vein

D. peroneal vein

8. Which of the following does **not** lie in the malleolar canal? (   )

A. Tendon of tibialis posterior

B. Tendon of flexor digitorum longus

C. Deep peroneal nerve

D. Posterior tibial vessels

II. Double choices (Choose the two best answers among the following answers, and write the corresponding letters in the bracket)

1. The flexor retinaculum lies between two structures, they are (   ).

A. medial malleolus

B. lateral malleolus

C. calcaneus

D. talus

E. medial border of foot

2. The deep plantar arch is formed by the union of (   ).

A. dorsal metatarsal artery

B. deep plantar artery

C. arcuate artery

D. medial plantar artery

E. lateral plantar artery

3. The peroneal retinacula hold the tendon of (   ).

A. tibialis anterior

B. flexor digitorum longus

C. extensor digitorum longus

D. peroneus longus

E. peroneus brevis

4. The two terminal branches of the posterior tibial artery are (   ).

A. dorsal metatarsal artery

B. deep plantar artery

C. arcuate artery

D. medial plantar artery

E. lateral plantar artery

III. Fill the blanks (Fill the most appropriate words and phrases in the blanks)

1. The malleolar canal is formed by _____ , _____ and _____ .

2. From anterior posteriorly, the structures passing through the malleolar canal are ____ _____ , _____ , _____ and _____ .

3. The terminal branches of posterior tibial artery are _____ and _____ .

4. On the sole of foot, tibial nerve divides into _____ and _____ .

5. The inferior extensor retinaculum forms three osseofibrous tunnels for holding the tendons of _____ , _____ and _____ .

IV. Answer the questions briefly

1. Briefly describe the cutaneous nerves of the dorsum of foot.

2. Briefly describe the formation and contents of the malleolar canal.

Chapter 5　The Thorax

Section 1　Introduction

Outline and Objectives

Ⅰ. Grasp

The main surface landmarks, marking lines and their clinical significance and understand the boundaries of the thorax.

Ⅱ. Comprehend

The boundaries and divisions of the thorax.

Exercises

Ⅰ. Single choice (Choose the best answer among the following four answers, and write the corresponding letter in the bracket)

About the sternal angle, which of the following descriptions is correct? (　　)

A. The sternal angle is opposite to the upper border of the 4th thoracic vertebra.

B. The sternal angle marks the surface projection of the bifurcation of the trachea.

C. The sternal angle marks the level of the origin of the aortic arch from the descending aorta.

D. The sternal angle marks the level of the first physiological constriction of the esophagus.

Ⅱ. Double choices (Choose the two best answers among the following answers, and write the corresponding letters in the bracket)

Which of the following are at the level of sternal angle? (　　)

A. thymus

B. esophageal hiatus

C. bifurcation of trachea

D. pulmonary artery

E. lower border of the 4th thoracic vertebra

Ⅲ. Fill the blanks (Fill the most appropriate words and phrases in the blanks)

The costal margin (costal arch) is formed by the ＿＿＿＿＿costal cartilages.

Section 2   The Thoracic Wall

Outline and Objectives

Ⅰ. Grasp

1. The superficial structures of the thoracic wall and the proper composition of it.
2. The location, structure, blood supply and the lymphatic drainage of female breast of the female breast.
3. The composition of intercostal space, the relationship of posterior intercostal blood vessels and intercostal nerves, and the site of pleural cavity puncture and its clinical significance.
4. The course and branches of internal thoracic artery.

Ⅱ. Comprehend

1. The layers of the thoracic wall.
2. The distribution of superficial and deep fascia and muscle in the thoracic wall.

Exercises

Ⅰ. Single choice (Choose the best answer among the following four answers, and write the corresponding letter in the bracket)

1. The following structures constitute the female breast, **except** (　　).

   A. the fatty tissue

   B. the skin

   C. the mammary gland

   D. the smooth muscle

2. Which of the following statements about the position of the female breast is **not** true? (　　)

   A. The female breast overlies the 2nd to the 6th ribs.

   B. It is located in the deep fascia of the thoracic wall.

   C. It extends laterally to the midaxillary line.

   D. It extends medially to the parasternal line.

3. Which of the following statements about the female breast is true? (　　)

   A. The mammary glands lie in the pectoralis fascia.

   B. The lobules consist of a cluster of alveoli opens into the lactiferous ducts.

   C. The lateral part of the female breast is supplied by the internal thoracicartery.

   D. Its medial lymphatic vessels drain into the pectoral lymph nodes.

4. Which of the following is related to the orange-peel type skin lesions of the female breast? (　　)

 A. The fatty tissue

 B. The Cooper's ligaments

 C. The lactiferous ducts

 D. The areolar glands

5. Which of the following raises the rib and assist in inspiration? (　　)

 A. The intercostales externi

 B. The intercostales interni

 C. The intercostales intimi

 D. The serratus anterior

6. Which of the following supplies blood for the medial part of the female breast? (　　)

 A. The posterior intercostal artery

 B. The lateral thoracic artery

 C. The thoracoacromial artery

 D. The internal thoracic artery

7. Which of the following statements about the posterior intercostal artery is **wrong**? (　　)

 A. There are 11 pairs of posterior intercostal arteries totally.

 B. The subcostal artery arises from the lumbar artery.

 C. The costocervical trunk and superior thoracic artery supply for the area of the first and second intercostal spaces.

 D. The eleven pairs of posterior intercostal arteries arise from the thoracic aorta.

8. Which of the following statements about the internal thoracic artery is true? (　　)

 A. It arises from the axillary artery.

 B. Its perforating branches supply blood for the medial part of the female breast.

 C. Its terminal branches are the superior epigastric and pericardiacophrenic arteries.

 D. Its musculophrenic artery accompanies the phrenic nerve.

9. Which of the following drains into the pectoral lymph nodes? (　　)

 A. The lymphatic vessels of medial part of the female breast

 B. The lymphatic vessels of the inferior part of the female breast

 C. The lymphatic vessels of the lateral part of the female breast

 D. The apical lymph nodes

10. Which of the following about the intercostal nerve is **not** true? (　　)

 A. There are twelve pairs of intercostal nerves.

 B. The 3rd to 6th intercostal nerves control the sensation of female breast.

 C. The 7th to 11th intercostal nerves supply the thoracic wall andabdominal wall.

 D. The intercostal nerve arises from the ventral rami of the thoracic spinal nerve.

II. Double choices (Choose the two best answers among the following answers, and write the corresponding letters in the bracket)

1. Which ones of the following supply blood for the female breast? (   )

   A. The perforating branches of the internal thoracic artery

   B. The lateral thoracic artery

   C. The perforating branches of posterior intercostal artery

   D. The subcostal artery

   E. The subclavian artery

2. Which ones of the following about the intercostal space are true? (   )

   A. There are three layers of the muscles in each intercostal space.

   B. The external intercostal membrane is superficial to the intercostales externi.

   C. The internal intercostal membrane is deep to the intercostales interni.

   D. In the costal groove of the rib, the posterior intercostal vein lies at the top.

   E. There are anastomoses between the internal thoracic artery and posterior intercostal artery in each intercostal space.

3. Which of the following statements about the female breast are **not** true? (   )

   A. It is composed of skin, fatty tissue and mammary glands.

   B. It lies superficial to the pectoralis fascia.

   C. It extends laterally to the anterior axillary line.

   D. The medial part of the female breast is supplied by the internal thoracic artery.

   E. Its medial lymphatic vessels drain into the pectoral lymph nodes.

4. Which of the following pass through the clavipectoral fascia? (   )

   A. lateral thoracic artery

   B. superior thoracic artery

   C. cephalic vein

   D. lateral pectoral nerve

   E. axillary nerve

5. Which of the following statements about the intercostal nerve are **not** true? (   )

   A. There are 11 pairs of intercostal nerves totally.

   B. It gives off the medial and lateral pectoral nerves.

   C. It runs between the intercostales externi and the intercostales interni.

   D. It has cutaneous and muscular branches.

   E. Its anterior cutaneous branches emerge from 1 – 2 cm lateral to the margin of the sternum.

III. Fill the blanks (Fill the most appropriate words and phrases in the blanks)

1. There are the _____ , _____ , _____ and _____ four structures passing through the clavipectoral fascia which extends between the subclavius and the upper border of the pectoralis minor.

2. In the costal groove of the ribs, the arrangement from up downwards is the _____ , _____ , and _____ .

IV. Answer the questions briefly

1. Briefly describe the clavipectoral fascia.
2. Briefly describe the structures of the intercostal space from the costal angel to the costochondral junction.
3. Briefly describe the position and structures of the female breast.

V. Answer the questions in detail

1. Describe the lymphatic drainage of the female breast.
2. Describe the cutaneous nerves of the anterior thoracic wall.

Section 3   The Pleura, Pleural Cavity and Lungs

Outline and Objectives

I. Grasp

1. The subdivision of the pleura and the construction of the pleural cavity and the position of the pleural recess.
2. The surface projection of the refraction line of the parietal pleura, and the location and clinical significance of pericardial triangle.
3. The position of the lungs, the composition and arrangement of lung roots, and the adjacent relation of lung roots.

II. Comprehend

The concepts, characteristics and clinical significance of bronchus, pulmonary lobe, bronchopulmonary segments, principal bronchia and the trachea.

Exercises

I. Single choice (Choose the best answer among the following four answers, and write the corresponding letter in the bracket)

1. Which of the following statements about pleura is **not** true? (   )
   A. It is a layer of serous membrane.
   B. It has parietal and visceral two parts.
   C. The visceral pleura can be divided into four parts.
   D. The cupula of the pleura extends into the root of the neck.
2. Which of the following statements about pleural cavity is true? (   )
   A. The pleural cavity is enclosed by the parietal pleura.

    B. There is only a little serous fluid and air in the pleural cavity.

    C. There are two pleural cavities communicating with each other.

    D. The pleural cavity presents a negative pressure.

3. Which of the following statements about pleural recesses is true? (　　)

    A. The pleural recesses are formed by the reflection of the visceral pleura.

    B. The pleural recesses are formed by the reflection of the parietal pleura.

    C. The largest pleural recess is the costomediastinal recess.

    D. The pleural recesses can be occupied by the expand lung at deep inspiration.

4. Which of the following is the lowest part of the pleural cavity at an upright or seated position? (　　)

    A. The costomediastinal recess

    B. The cupula

    C. The mediastinal pleura

    D. The costodiaphragmatic recess

5. Which of the following statements about the lower border of pleura is **not** true? (　　)

    A. It lies at the horizontal level of the 10th rib in the midaxillary line.

    B. It lies at the horizontal level of the 11th rib in the scapular line.

    C. On the left side, it commences from the back of the 6th sternocostal joint.

    D. It lies at the horizontal level of the 8th rib in the midclavicular line.

6. Which of the following statements about the root of the lung is true? (　　)

    A. The root of the lung is form by the structures passing through the hilum of the lung enclosed by the pleura.

    B. The vagus nerve lies in front of the root of the lung.

    C. The aortic arch lies above the root of the lung on the right side.

    D. The azygos vein arch lies above the root of the lung on the left side.

7. Which of the following statements about the lung is true? (　　)

    A. The left lung has three lobes.

    B. There is a cardiac notch at the anterior border of the right lung.

    C. The inferior pulmonary vein lies at the most lower part of the hilum.

    D. The bronchus lies at the front of the root of the lung.

8. Which of the following statements about the pulmonary ligament is true? (　　)

    A. It is formed by a single layer of pleura.

    B. It present at coronal position.

    C. It extends between the lung and diaphragm.

    D. It is a part of the root of the lung.

9. Which of the following is the most likely to be injured by mistake in a surgery at the root of neck? (　　)

    A. The costal pleura

    B. The pulmonary vein

C. The pulmonary artery

D. The cupula of pleura

10. Which of the following belongs to two layers of pleura? (   )

    A. The pulmonary ligament

    B. The mediastinal pleura

    C. The endothoracic fascia

    D. The cupula of pleura

II . Double choices (Choose the two best answers among the following answers, and write the corresponding letters in the bracket)

1. Which of the following lie in front of the root lung? (   )

    A. The phrenic nerve

    B. The azygos vein

    C. The vagus nerve

    D. The pulmonary ligament

    E. The pericardiacophrenic vessels

2. Which of the following statements about the pleura are true? (   )

    A. The cupula is continuous with visceral pleura.

    B. The lower border of the pleura commences from the back of the 6th sternocostal joint on the right side.

    C. The lower border of the pleura commences from the back of the midpoint of the 6th costal cartilage on the left side.

    D. The pulmonary ligament is formed by the visceral pleura.

    E. The root of the lung is enclosed by parietal pleura.

3. Which of the following statements about costodiaphragmatic recess are true? (   )

    A. It is the lowest part of the pleural cavity.

    B. It is formed by the reflection of the parietal and visceral pleura.

    C. It is formed by reflection of the mediastinal pleura and the costal pleura.

    D. It is a common puncture site of pleural effusion in clinic.

    E. It only exists on the left side.

4. Which of the following are formed by reflections of parietal and visceral pleura? (   )

    A. The endothoracic fascia

    B. The pulmonary ligament

    C. The pleural cavity

    D. The costodiaphragmatic recess

    E. The cupula of pleura

5. Which of the following statements about the hilum of the lung are true? (   )

    A. The bronchus lies in the most front of the pulmonary hilum.

    B. The pulmonary artery lies in the most front of the pulmonary hilum.

C. The structures passing through the hilum of the lung are surrounded by the pleura.

D. The hilum of the lung lies near the center of the costal surface.

E. The inferior pulmonary vein is located at lowest of the pulmonary hilum.

III. Fill the blanks (Fill the most appropriate words and phrases in the blanks)

1. The chief structures passing through the hilum of each lung from anterior to the posterior are the _____ , _____ and _____ .

2. The chief structures passing through the hilum of the right lung from above downwards are the _____ , _____ , _____ and _____ .

3. The two parts of the pleura are the _____ and _____ .

4. The lowest portion of the pleural cavity is the _____ .

5. The distance between the anterior borders of both pleura below the level of the 4th costal cartilage is named _____ .

IV. Answer the questions briefly

1. Briefly describe the pleura and parietal pleura.

2. Briefly describe the pleural cavity and pleural recesses.

3. Briefly describe the chief structures enclosed in the root of lung.

4. Briefly describe the lower border of the pleura.

5. Briefly describe relations of the root of the lung.

V. Answer the questions in detail

1. Describe the surface projections of the reflections of pleura.

2. Describe the position, external features, lobes of the lungs, and the arrangement of the chief structures passing through the hilum of the lungs.

Section 4   The Diaphragm

Outline and Objectives

I. Grasp

1. The location and division of diaphragm.

2. The openings of diaphragm and the structures passing through the openings.

II. Comprehend

The triangles of the diaphragm.

Exercises

Ⅰ. **Single choice（Choose the best answer among the following four answers, and write the corresponding letter in the bracket）**

1. Which of the following statements about diaphragm is **not** true? (   )

   A. The diaphragm is a dome-shaped septum separating the thoracic cavity from the abdominal cavity.

   B. The diaphragm can be divided into the central tendon and the peripheral muscular part.

   C. Its muscular fibers consist of the sternal, costal and lumbar three parts.

   D. The esophagus hiatus is located in the central tendon.

2. Which of the following passes through the aortic hiatus? (   )

   A. The vagus nerve

   B. The thoracic duct

   C. The phrenic nerve

   D. The right lymphatic duct

Ⅱ. **Double choices（Choose the two best answers among the following answers, and write the corresponding letters in the bracket）**

1. Which of the following do not pass through the openings of the diaphragm? (   )

   A. The vagus nerve

   B. The hepatic portal vein

   C. The phrenic nerve

   D. The thoracic duct

   E. The right lymphatic duct

2. Which of the following statements about diaphragm are true? (   )

   A. Its muscular fibers arise from the margin of the thoracic outlet and front of the bodies of the upper 3 lumbar vertebrae.

   B. The aorta and the thoracic duct transmit the aortic hiatus.

   C. The esophageal hiatus is located 2 – 3 cm to the right of the median plane.

   D. The vena caval foramen is located at the level of the 10th thoracic vertebra.

   E. Its muscular portion is divided into costal and lumbar two parts.

Ⅲ. **Fill the blanks（Fill the most appropriate words and phrases in the blanks）**

1. The muscular fibers of diaphragm are divided into _____, _____ and _____ three parts.

2. The aortic hiatus is at the level of _____ thoracic vertebra, slightly to the left of the median plane. The aorta, _____ and _____ transmit the hiatus.

IV. **Answer the questions briefly**

Briefly describe the openings of the diaphragm and the structures passing through them.

Section 5   The Mediastinum

Outline and Objectives

I. Grasp

1. The left and right view of the mediastinum.

2. The division of mediastinum, the layers and contents of superior mediastinum.

3. The position, boundaries contents (the left recurrent laryngeal nerve, superficial cardiac plexus and the arterial ligament) of triangle of ductus arteriosus and its clinical significance.

4. The position, relation, blood supply and lymphatic drainage of the thoracic part of the esophagus.

5. The adjacent relationship and clinical significance of heart, thoracic duct and thoracic aorta.

II. Comprehend

1. The arrangement of trachea, esophagus, thoracic duct, vagus nerve and phrenic nerve.

2. The position and relation of pericardial sinus and its clinical significance.

3. The course of the azygos vein, hemiazygos vein and their relationship with esophageal vein.

Exercises

I. Single choice (Choose the best answer among the following four answers, and write the corresponding letter in the bracket)

1. Which of the following lies in the middle layer of the superior mediastinum? (   )

   A. The thymus

   B. The left brachiocephalic vein

   C. The superior vena cava

   D. The left phrenic nerve

2. Which of the following is **not** located in the posterior mediastinum? (   )

   A. The thoracic aorta

   B. The trachea

   C. The esophagus

   D. The hemiazygos vein

3. Which of the following is a landmark on the left side of the mediastinum in a pos-
   teroanterior chest radiograph? (   )
   A. The terminal portion of the aortic arch
   B. The origin of the ascending aorta
   C. The origin of the thoracic aorta
   D. The azygos arch

4. Which of the following supplys blood for the superior esophagus? (   )
   A. The thoracic aorta
   B. The internal thoracic artery
   C. The bronchial artery
   D. The subclavian artery

5. The second physiological constriction of the esophagus lies at (   ).
   A. the part behind the left principal bronchus
   B. the part behind the bronchial bifurcation
   C. the part behind the thoracic aorta
   D. the part behind the right principal bronchus

6. Which of the following lies in the anterior mediastinum? (   )
   A. The pericardium
   B. The anterior lymph nodes
   C. The phrenic nerve
   D. The superficial cardiac plexuses

7. Which of the following lies left to the superior vena cava? (   )
   A. The azygos vein
   B. The trachea and vagus nerve
   C. The right phrenic nerve
   D. The ascending aorta and aortic arch

8. Which of the following lies in the ductus arteriosus triangle? (   )
   A. The left phrenic nerve
   B. The left vagus nerve
   C. The left recurrent laryngeal nerve
   D. The left pulmonary artery

9. The thoracic aorta is continuous with the aortic arch at the level of lower border of
   (   ).
   A. the second thoracic vertebra
   B. the third thoracic vertebra
   C. the fourth thoracic vertebra
   D. the fifth thoracic vertebra

10. Which of the following statements about the thoracic part of the esophagus is **not** true? ( )

 A. It lies in the posterior mediastinum.

 B. It passes through the esophageal hiatus to enter abdomen.

 C. The superior segment lies right to the thoracic aorta.

 D. The inferior segment lies left to the thoracic aorta.

11. Which of the following lies behind the pericardium? ( )

 A. The esophagus

 B. The superior vena cava

 C. The mediastinal pleura

 D. The central tendon of the diaphragm

12. Which of the following lies right to the thoracic part of the esophagus? ( )

 A. The trachea

 B. The pericardium

 C. The superior vena cava

 D. The arch of azygos vein

13. The azygos vein commences as the continuation of the ( ).

 A. hemiazygos vein

 B. right ascending lumbar vein

 C. accessory hemiazygos vein

 D. left ascending lumbar vein

14. The thoracic duct begins at the ( ).

 A. left lumbar trunk

 B. intestinal trunk

 C. cisterna chyli

 D. left bronchomediastinal trunk

15. The thoracic duct ends by opening into the ( ).

 A. left venous angle

 B. left subclavian vein

 C. right venous angle

 D. right jugular vein

Ⅱ. Double choices (Choose the two best answers among the following answers, and write the corresponding letters in the bracket)

1. The phrenic nerve descends ( ).

 A. in front of the root of lung

 B. behind the subclavian vein

 C. behind the root of lung

 D. behind the scalenus anterior

 E. behind the subclavian artery

2. The branches of the aortic arch do **not** include (   ).

   A. the brachiocephalic trunk

   B. the left common carotid artery

   C. the internal thoracic artery

   D. the left subclavian artery

   E. coronary artery

3. Which of the following do **not** belong to the direct tributaries of the superior vena cava? (   )

   A. The left brachiocephalic vein

   B. The internal jugular vein

   C. The azygos vein

   D. The subclavian vein

   E. The right brachiocephalic vein

4. Which of the following statements about the thoracic duct are true? (   )

   A. It is formed by the union of the left lumbar trunk, right lumbar trunk and intestinal trunk.

   B. It origins from the cisterna chyli.

   C. It passes obliquely behind the esophagus to reach its right side at the level of the lower border of the 4th thoracic vertebrae.

   D. It passed through the esophageal hiatus to enter the thoracic cavity.

   E. It only receives the lymph of the left jugular trunk, subclavian trunk and bronchomediastinal trunk.

5. Which of the following are **not** located in the posterior mediastinum? (   )

   A. The vagus nerve

   B. The trachea

   C. The aortic arch

   D. The thoracic duct

   E. The greater splanchnic nerve

6. Which of the following lie in the middle layer of the superior mediastinum? (   )

   A. The vagus nerve

   B. The thoracic duct

   C. The trachea

   D. The left subclavian artery

   E. The superior vane cava

7. The following structures lie anterior to thoracic aorta, **except** (   ).

   A. the root of the left lung

   B. the pericardium

   C. the esophagus

   D. the trachea

   E. the thoracic duct

8. The veins of the esophagus would **not** join into (   ).

A. the hepatic portal vein

B. the azygos vein

C. the right jugular vein

D. the hemiazygos vein

E. the subclavian vein

Ⅲ. Fill the blanks (Fill the most appropriate words and phrases in the blanks)

1. The brachiocephalic vein is formed by the union of the _____ and _____ .

2. The aortic arch given off three branches from its convexity, they are _____ , __ _____ and _____ .

3. The thoracic part of sympathetic trunk consists of 10 – 12 ganglia, among them the 5th – 9th ganglia send branches to form the _____ which enters the abdomen and goes to the celiac ganglion.

4. The thoracicduct arises from the _____ which lies in front of the first and second lumbar vertebrae.

5. At the level of 4th thoracic vertebra, the azygos arch strides across the _____ anteriorly and then join the _____ .

Ⅳ. Answer the questions briefly

1. Briefly describe the layers of the superior mediastinum and the contents in each layer.

2. Briefly describe the boundary and contents of the ductus arteriosus triangle.

3. Briefly describe the relations of the thoracic part of the esophagus.

4. Briefly describe the location, contents and communications of the retroesophageal space.

Ⅴ. Answer the questions in detail

1. Describe the left view of the mediastinum.

2. Describe the location, relations, blood supply and lymphatic drainage of the thoracic part of the esophagus.

Chapter 6 The Abdomen

Section 1 Introduction

Outline and Objectives

Ⅰ. Grasp

1. The surface landmarks, reference lines of the abdomen.
2. The surface projections of the visceral organs such as liver, stomach, gallbladder, spleen, pancreas, vermiform appendix, small intestine, kidney, etc.

Ⅱ. Comprehend

1. The boundaries and nine regions divisions of the abdomen.

Exercises

Ⅰ. Single choice (Choose the best answer among the following four answers, and write the corresponding letter in the bracket)

1. The roof of the abdominal cavity is (　　).
   A. at the level of the twelfth thoracic vertebra
   B. at the level of the twelfth rib
   C. at the level of the xiphoid process
   D. diaphragm

2. Concerning the boundaries of the abdomen, which statement is correct? (　　)
   A. The 11th ribs do not form the superior boundaries.
   B. The posterior superior iliac spine does not form the inferior boundaries.
   C. The superior boundary of abdomen is also the inferior boundary of the thorax.
   D. The superior boundary of the abdominal wall is the same as the superior boundary of the abdominal cavity.

3. Which of the following organs is **not** located in the right lumbar region? (　　)
   A. The lower part of the right kidney
   B. The upper part of the right kidney
   C. Ascending colon
   D. Part of ileum

II. Double choices (Choose the two best answers among the following answers, and write the corresponding letters in the bracket)

1. The lower horizontal line dividing the abdominal cavity into 9 regions may pass through (　　).

  A. anterior superior iliac spine

  B. anterior inferior iliac spine

  C. iliac crest

  D. iliac tubercle

  E. umbilicus

2. The vertical line dividing the abdominal cavity into 9 regions passes through (　　).

  A. midclavicular line

  B. pubic tubercle

  C. midpoint of inguinal ligament

  D. iliac tubercle

  E. umbilicus

3. The left inguinal region includes (　　).

  A. cecum

  B. vermiform appendix

  C. sigmoid colon

  D. descending colon

  E. ileum

III. Fill the blanks (Fill the most appropriate words and phrases in the blanks)

1. The abdomen consists of _____ , _____ and _____ .

2. The superior boundary of abdominal cavity is _____ ; its inferior boundary is _____ .

3. The lateral border of rectus abdominis and its sheath is indicated by the _____ on surface.

4. The level of the umbilicus passes through between the _____ and _____ lumbar vertebrae.

5. About 2.5 cm above the umbilicus, _____ artery originates from the abdominal aorta.

Section 2　The Anterolateral Abdominal Wall

Outline and Objectives

I. Grasp

1. The positions, shapes, origins, insertions and actions of the anterolateral group mus-

cles (obliquus externus abdominis, obliquus internus abdominis, transversus abdominis and rectus abdominis).

2. The layers of the anterolateral wall and their characteristics.

3. The distribution of the blood vessels and nerves in deep layer of the anterolateral wall.

4. The constitute and feature of the sheath of rectus abdominis.

5. The position, constitute (superior wall, inferior wall, anterior wall, posterior wall, and two openings), projection and contents (spermatic cord in male, round ligament of uterus in female and the accompanying nerves) of the inguinal canal.

Ⅱ. Comprehend

1. The feature of the skin of abdomen and the structural characteristic, the drainage of the superficial vein and the distribution of the cutaneous nerve of the superficialfascia of anterolateral wall of the abdomen.

2. The position, features (central tendon and three openings) of the diaphragm.

3. The anatomical basis of the inguinal hernias and difference between the direct inguinal hernia and the indirect inguinal hernia.

Exercises

Ⅰ. Single choice (Choose the best answer among the following four answers, and write the corresponding letter in the bracket)

1. Which incision does **not** meet muscle during abdominal operation? (   )

    A. Median incision

    B. Paramedian incision

    C. Subcostal incision

    D. McBurney's incision

2. About the skin of anterolateral abdominal wall, which statement is **incorrect**? (   )

    A. It is thin and elastic.

    B. It is movable except the umbilicus.

    C. Its sensation has no segmental characteristic.

    D. The skin in inguinal region is usually chosen for implantation.

3. Which of the following statements about Scarpa fascia is correct? (   )

    A. It is alsoregarded as a fatty layer.

    B. It is more superficial than Camper fascia.

    C. It is continuous with anterior sheath of the rectus abdominis medially.

    D. It is membranous.

4. The intercostal nerve distributed in the level of umbilicus is (   ).

    A. the sixth

    B. the eighth

C. the ninth

D. the tenth

5. About the superficial fascia of anterolateral abdominal wall, which statement is correct? (   )

A. It lacks fat.

B. It is lack of superficial artery.

C. There is a venous plexus around the umbilicus.

D. The whole lymph was drained into superficial inguinal lymph nodes.

6. Which vein does **not** belong to the superficial vein of the anterolateral abdominal wall?

(   )

A. Superficial epigastric vein

B. Superficial iliac circumflex vein

C. Thoracoepigastric vein

D. Inferior epigastric vein

7. The muscle just on each side of the anterior median line is (   ).

A. rectus abdominis

B. obliquus externus abdominis

C. obliquus internus abdominis

D. transversus abdominis

8. Which of the following statements about arcuate line is correct? (   )

A. It is alsoregarded as semicircular line.

B. It is on the lateral side of the rectus abdominis.

C. It is at the level of umbilicus.

D. It forms the superior wall of the inguinal canal.

9. The inguinal ligament is formed by (   ).

A. camper fascia

B. scapa fascia

C. aponeurosis of the obliquus externus abdominis

D. fascia lata

10. The internal spermatic fascia is formed by (   ).

A. aponeurosis of the obliquus externus abdominis

B. aponeurosis of the transversus abdominis

C. aponeurosis of the obliquus internus abdominis

D. transverse fascia

11. About the obliquus externus abdominis, which of the following statements is correct? (   )

A. The direction of its fibers is from medial to lateral.

B. It originates from inguinal ligament.

C. Its aponeurosis forms the superficial ring of the inguinal canal.

D. It inserts into the external surface of lower nine ribs.

12. About the obliquus internus abdominis, which of the following statement is correct?
    (   )
    A. The direction of its fibers is horizontal.
    B. Its aponeurosis takes part in the sheath of rectus abdominis.
    C. It originates from linea alba.
    D. It inserts into the inguinal ligament.

13. About the transversus abdominis, which of the following statement is correct? (   )
    A. It is superficial to the obliquus internus abdominis.
    B. It inserts into the internal surface of lower six ribs.
    C. Its aponeurosis forms the posterior wall of the inguinal canal.
    D. It forms a part of the cremaster.

14. The inguinal falx inserts to (   ).
    A. inguinal ligament
    B. pectineal ligament
    C. iliac crest
    D. linea alba

15. The cremaster is innervated by (   ).
    A. iliohypogastric nerve
    B. ilioinguinal nerve
    C. genitofemoral nerve
    D. obturator nerve

16. The artery arising from the femoral artery is (   ).
    A. inferior gastric artery
    B. superficial gastric artery
    C. deep iliac circumflex artery
    D. superior gastric artery

17. The artery that does not supply the abdominal wall is (   ).
    A. obturator artery
    B. superior gastric artery
    C. subcostal artery
    D. superior iliac circumflex artery

18. The structure lying between parietal peritoneum and transverse fascia is (   ).
    A. rectus abdominis
    B. extraperitoneal fascia
    C. transversus abdominis
    D. obliquus internus abdominis

19. The parietal peritoneum forms the following structures, **except** for (   ).
    A. median umbilical fold
    B. medial umbilical fold

C. posterior wall of inguinal canal

D. deep inguinal ring

20. The aponeurosis of obliquus externus abdominis forms the following structures,
   except for (　　).

   A. medial crus

   B. lateral crus

   C. inguinal ligament

   D. inguinal flax

21. The wall of inguinal canal formed by inguinal ligament is (　　).

   A. anterior wall

   B. posterior wall

   C. superior wall

   D. inferior wall

22. The inguinal triangle is bounded laterally by (　　).

   A. lateral border of rectus abdominis

   B. inferior epigastric artery

   C. deep iliac circumflex artery

   D. inguinal ligament

23. The deep inguinal ring is formed by (　　).

   A. transverse fascia

   B. extraperitoneal fascia

   C. transversus abdominis

   D. obliquus internus abdominis

24. The lateral umbilicus fold contains (　　).

   A. inferior epigastric vessels

   B. umbilical artery

   C. umbilical vein

   D. urachus

Ⅱ. Double choices (Choose the two best answers among the following answers, and write the corresponding letters in the bracket)

1. The structures formed by transverse fascia are (　　).

   A. pectineal ligament

   B. deep inguinal ring

   C. superficial inguinal ring

   D. lacunar ligament

   E. interfoveolar ligament

2. The anterior wall of inguinal canal is formed by (　　).

   A. inguinal ligament

B. aponeurosis of obliquus externus abdominis

C. transverse fascia

D. partial origin of obliquus internus abdominis

E. inferior border of transversus abdominis

3. The following structures are formed by the aponeurosis of obliquus externus abdominis, **except** for (   ).

A. inguinal ligament

B. superficial ring of inguinal canal

C. deep ring of inguinal canal

D. lateral crus

E. interfoveolar ligament

4. The fibers of cremaster come from (   ).

A. rectus abdominis

B. obliquus externus abdominis

C. obliquus internus abdominis

D. transversus abdominis

E. transverse fascia

5. The nerves passing through the inguinal canal are (   ).

A. femoral branch of genitofemoral nerve

B. genital branch of genitofemoral nerve

C. iliohypogastric nerve

D. ilioinguinal nerve

E. subcostal nerve

Ⅲ. Fill the blanks (Fill the most appropriate words and phrases in the blanks)

1. The superficial fascia of anterolateral abdominal wall below umbilicus consists of two layers: _____ and _____.

2. The nerve distributed in the level of xiphoid process is _____. The nerve distributed in the level of umbilicus is _____.

3. The superficial arteries supplying the lower part of anterolateral abdominal wall are _____ and _____. Both arise from _____.

4. The superficial vein above umbilicus converge to form _____, then drain the blood into _____ via lateral thoracic vein.

5. Below umbilicus, the blood flows through _____ and _____ into great saphenous vein.

6. The lymph above umbilicus is drained into _____; below umbilicus, it empties into _____.

7. The muscles of the anterolateral abdominal wall consist of _____, _____, _____ and _____.

8. The main structure passing through the male inguinal canal is _____ , while it is _____ in the female inguinal canal.

9. The arteries deep to rectus abdominis are _____ and _____ .

10. The Hesselbach triangle is bounded by _____ , _____ and _____ .

IV. Answer the questions briefly

1. Describe the usual incisions during abdominal operation.

2. Describe the layers of the lateral abdominal wall.

3. Describe the structures formed by the aponeurosis of obliquus externus abdominis.

4. Describe the arteries in the deep structure of the anterolateral abdominal wall.

V. Answer the questions in detail

1. Please describe the location, formation and contents in the inguinal canal. What is the clinical significance?

2. Please describe the sheath of the rectus abdominis.

Section 3　The Peritoneum and Peritoneal Cavity

Outline and Objectives

I. Grasp

1. The conception, division (parietal peritoneum and visceral peritoneum) and function of the peritoneum.

2. The conception, division (greater sac and lesser sac) and characteristic of peritoneal cavity.

3. The three kinds (intra-peritoneal organs, meso-peritoneal organs and extra-peritoneal organs) of the abdominal and pelvic viscera according to the relation between viscera and peritoneum.

4. The structures formed by the peritoneum such as ligaments, omenta and mesenteries.

5. The spaces of the supracolic compartment and the sulci and sinuses of the infracolic compartment.

II. Comprehend

1. The folds, recesses and pouches formed by the peritoneum and the communications of the intraperitoneal space.

2. The location, boundaries and communication of the omental bursa.

3. The boundaries of the omental foramen.

Exercises

Ⅰ. **Single choice（Choose the best answer among the following four answers，and write the corresponding letter in the bracket）**

 1. Which one of the following belongs to the meso-peritoneal organ? (　　)

  A. Stomach

  B. Liver

  C. Spleen

  D. Pancreas

 2. Which one of the following belongs to the intra-peritoneal organs? (　　)

  A. Duodenum

  B. Ileum

  C. Ascending colon

  D. Gallbladder

 3. Which one of the following belongs to the extra-peritoneal organ? (　　)

  A. Liver

  B. Uterus

  C. Kidney

  D. Spleen

 4. The lowest part of the peritoneal cavity in the male in the anatomical position is (　　).

  A. the omental bursa

  B. the rectovesical pouch

  C. the right paracolic sulcus

  D. the hepatorenal recess

 5. The lowest part of the peritoneal cavity in the supine position is (　　).

  A. the omental bursa

  B. the rectovesical pouch

  C. the left paracolic sulcus

  D. the hepatorenal recess

 6. Which of the following structures does **not** form the boundary of the omental foramen? (　　)

  A. Quadrate lobe of liver

  B. Hepatoduodenal ligament

  C. The inferior vena cava covered by peritoneum

  D. The superior part of duodenum

 7. Which of the following ligaments of liver is **not** formed by peritoneum? (　　)

  A. Falciform ligament

  B. Ligamentum teres hepatis

  C. Hepatogastric ligament

  D. Coronary ligament

8. Which of the following statements about peritoneum is **incorrect**? (   )

   A. It consists of the parietal peritoneum and visceral peritoneum.

   B. The peritoneal cavity is enclosed by the peritoneal and parietal peritoneum.

   C. It is a serous membrane.

   D. It has no function to excrete substance.

9. The layer of peritoneum in lesser omentum is (   ).

   A. 1   B. 2   C. 3   D. 4

10. The layer of peritoneum in lower partof greater omentum is (   ).

    A. 1   B. 2   C. 3   D. 4

Ⅱ. **Double choices (Choose the two best answers among the following answers, and write the corresponding letters in the bracket)**

1. The extra-peritoneal organ includes (   ).

   A. kidney   B. uterus   C. ureter   D. ovary   E. gallbladder

2. Which of the following structures formed by peritoneum contain blood vessels? (   )

   A. Median umbilical fold

   B. Lateral umbilical fold

   C. Suspensory ligament of ovary

   D. Proper ligament of ovary

   E. Ligamentum teres hepatis

3. The following structures are formed by the peritoneum, **except** for (   ).

   A. round ligament of uterus

   B. broad ligament of uterus

   C. uterosacral ligament of uterus

   D. cardinal ligament of uterus

   E. suspensory ligament of ovary

4. Which of the following organs have **no** mesentery? (   )

   A. Transverse colon

   B. Descending colon

   C. Sigmoid colon

   D. Jejunum

   E. Duodenum

5. Which of the following spaces belong to the infracolic compartment? (   )

   A. Right subhepatic space

   B. Omental bursa

   C. Paracolic sulcus

   D. Rectovesical pouch

   E. Mesenteric sinus

Ⅲ. Fill the blanks (Fill the most appropriate words and phrases in the blanks)

1. The structures formed by peritoneum include _____ , _____ and _____ .

2. The lesser omentum consists of _____ and _____ .

3. The lowest part of the peritoneal cavity in supine position is _____ .

4. The communication between greater sac and lesser sac is _____ .

5. Based on the covering of the peritoneum, the organs in abdominal cavity and pelvic cavity can be divided into _____ , _____ and _____ .

Ⅳ. Answer the questions briefly

1. Describe the location and the boundaries of the omental bursa.

2. Describe the ligaments formed by the peritoneum in supracolic compartment.

3. Describe the three groups of organs in abdominal cavity based on the covering of the peritoneum.

Ⅴ. Answer the questions in detail

Please describe the division and space of the peritoneal cavity.

Section 4   The Supracolic Compartment

Outline and Objectives

Ⅰ. Grasp

1. The division, position, relation, ligaments, blood vessels, lymphatic drainage and nerves of the stomach.

2. The position, shape, division and relations of the duodenum.

3. The shape, position and relation, ligaments, the porta hepatis and hepatic pedicle of the liver.

4. The constitute of extrahepatic biliary apparatus, the shape, division, position of the gallbladder, cystic duct, hepatic duct, common hepatic duct, and the division and relation of the common bile duct.

5. The location, boundaries and significance of the Calot triangle.

6. The shape, position and relation of the pancreas.

7. The shape, position, blood vessels and ligaments of the spleen.

8. The branches, course and distribution of the celiac trunk.

Ⅱ. Comprehend

1. The structures of the inner surface of the stomach.

2. The lobes, Glisson system and the segments of the liver.

3. Variations of the cystic artery.

Exercises

I . Single choice (Choose the best answer among the following four answers, and write the corresponding letter in the bracket)

1. Which organ does **not** lie in the supracolic compartment? (   )

    A. Stomach

    B. Liver

    C. Spleen

    D. Suprarenal gland

2. About the abdominal part of esophagus, which statement is **incorrect**? (   )

    A. It is the shortest part of esophagus.

    B. It is located in the esophageal notch of the liver.

    C. Its veins drain into the azygous vein.

    D. The arteries supplying blood to it are the branches of the inferior phrenic artery and left gastric artery.

3. Which of the following statements about stomach is **incorrect**? (   )

    A. It is one part of the lower digestive canal.

    B. It is located in the left hypochondriac and epigastric regions.

    C. It is divided into 4 parts.

    D. Cardiac orifice is on the left of the 11th thoracic vertebra.

4. The left gastric artery arises from (   ).

    A. splenic artery

    B. common hepatic artery

    C. celiac trunk

    D. proper hepatic artery

5. Which organ does **not** form the "stomach bed"? (   )

    A. Spleen

    B. Pancreas

    C. Left kidney

    D. Right kidney

6. The veins along the lesser curvatureof stomach directly drain into (   ).

    A. hepatic portal vein

    B. splenic vein

    C. superior mesenteric vein

    D. inferior mesenteric vein

7. The lymph of the abdominal part of esophagus is drained into (   ).

    A. suprapyloric lymph nodes

    B. subpyloric lymph nodes

    C. left gastric lymph nodes

    D. right gastric lymph nodes

8. The lymph of the fundus of stomach is drained into (   ).

    A. suprapyloric lymph nodes

    B. left gastroepiploic lymph nodes

    C. left gastric lymph nodes

    D. splenic lymph nodes

9. The major duodenal papilla opens into (   ).

    A. the superior part of duodenum

    B. the descending part of duodenum

    C. the horizontal part of duodenum

    D. the ascending part of duodenum

10. The superior mesenteric artery is anteriorly to (   ).

    A. the superior part of duodenum

    B. the descending part of duodenum

    C. the horizontal part of duodenum

    D. the ascending part of duodenum

11. About the relationship of the duodenum, which of the following statements is cor-
    rect? (   )

    A. There are gallbladder, hepatic portal vein and inferior vena cava posteriorly of the
       superior part.

    B. The descending part is medially adjacent to the head of pancreas, common bile
       duct and right ureters, etc.

    C. The anterior and left surfaces of ascending part are covered by peritoneum.

    D. The ascending part ends at the left of the 3rd lumbar vertebra.

12. The right lobe of liver is separated from left lobe by (   ).

    A. coronary ligament

    B. ligamentum teres hepatis

    C. triangular ligament

    D. falciform ligament.

13. Cancer in head of pancreas usually results in blockage of bile at (   ).

    A. the first part of the common bile duct

    B. the second part of the common bile duct

    C. the third part of the common bile duct

    D. the fourth part of the common bile duct

14. The structure passing through the second porta hepatis is (   ).

    A. hepatic duct

    B. hepatic portal vein

    C. proper hepatic artery

    D. hepatic vein

15. Which of the following structures does **not** bound the Calot triangle? (　　)

A. Common bile duct

B. Common hepatic duct

C. Cystic duct

D. Inferior surface of liver

16. The visceral surface of liver is **not** adjacent to (　　).

A. right kidney

B. stomach

C. spleen

D. gallbladder

17. The hepatic portal vein is formed behind of (　　).

A. the head of pancreas

B. the neck of pancreas

C. the body of pancreas

D. the tail of pancreas

18. Which artery does **not** supply the pancreas? (　　)

A. Superior pancreaticoduodenal artery

B. Inferior pancreaticoduodenal artery

C. Splenic artery

D. Right gastric artery

19. The splenic notch is located on (　　).

A. superior border

B. inferior border

C. anterior surface

D. posterior surface

20. The splenic artery can be found in (　　).

A. gastrosplenic ligament

B. lienorenal ligament

C. phrenicosplenic ligament

D. ileocolic ligament

Ⅱ. **Double choices (Choose the two best answers among the following answers, and write the corresponding letters in the bracket)**

1. Which organs do **not** form the "stomach bed"? (　　)

A. Pancreas

B. Right kidney

C. Spleen

D. Duodenum

E. Transverse colon

2. Which arteries are **not** given from the splenic artery? (　　)

 A. Left gastric artery

 B. Left gastroepiploic artery

 C. Short gastric artery

 D. Posterior gastric artery

 E. Right gastroepiploic artery

3. The first porta hepatis does **not** contain (　　).

 A. hepatic duct

 B. hepatic vein

 C. branches of hepatic portal vein

 D. branches of proper hepatic artery

 E. branches of cystic artery

4. The arteries inside the lesser curvature of stomach are (　　).

 A. left gastric artery

 B. right gastric artery

 C. right gastroepiploic artery

 D. left gastroepiploic artery

 E. short gastric artery

5. The nerves passing through the esophageal hiatus are (　　).

 A. anterior vagal trunk

 B. posterior vagal trunk

 C. left phrenic nerve

 D. right phrenic nerve

 E. left sympathetic trunk

6. The hepatic portal vein is formed by union of (　　).

 A. superior mesenteric vein

 B. inferior mesenteric vein

 C. splenic vein

 D. left gastric vein

 E. right gastric vein

7. The gallbladder is inferiorly and posteriorly adjacent to (　　).

 A. stomach

 B. lesser omentum

 C. transverse colon

 D. right colic flexure

 E. duodenum

8. The hepatopancreatic ampulla is formed by union of (　　).

 A. hepatic duct

 B. cystic duct

C. common bile duct

D. pancreatic duct

E. accessory pancreatic duct

9. The splenic vein collects (   ).

　　A. superior mesenteric vein

　　B. inferior mesenteric vein

　　C. left gastroepiploic vein

　　D. left gastric vein

　　E. right gastric vein

10. The pancreas is located in (   ).

　　A. right hypochondriac region

　　B. left hypochondriac region

　　C. umbilical region

　　D. left lumbar region

　　E. epigastric region

Ⅲ. Fill the blanks (Fill the most appropriate words and phrases in the blanks)

1. The arteries distributed to the greater curvature of stomach are _____ and ____

　　_____.

2. The stomach receives both _____ and _____ nerves.

3. The anterior wall of stomach is behind _____, _____ and _____.

4. The flexure between the superior part and descending part of duodenum is _____

　　__; the flexure between the superior part and horizontal part of duodenum is _____

　　____; the boundary between duodenum and jejunum is _____.

5. Below umbilicus, the blood flows through _____ and _____ into great saphenous vein.

6. There are _____ and _____ in front of the horizontal part of duodenum.

7. The left longitudinal groove of liver is formed by union of _____ and _____

　　__; the right one is formed by union of _____ and _____.

8. The triangle of Calot is bounded by _____, _____ and _____.

9. The gallbladder is divided into _____, _____, _____ and _____.

10. The hepatopancreatic ampulla opens into duodenum via _____.

11. The concavity of duodenum encloses the _____ of pancreas.

12. The accessory pancreatic duct opens on the _____.

13. The important palpable diagnostic landmark of spleen is _____.

14. The splenic artery arises from _____, and runs to left, near the upper border of

　　_____.

15. The ligaments of spleeninclude _____, _____ and _____.

IV. Answer the questions briefly

1. Describe the porta hepatis.

2. Describe the location and relationship of the spleen.

3. Describe the location and division of the duodenum.

V. Answer the questions in detail

1. Please describe extrahepatic bile duct.

2. Please describe location, relationship, blood supply, lymphatic drainage and nerve innervation of the stomach.

Section 5   The Infracolic Compartment

Outline and Objectives

I. Grasp

1. The locations, shapes, blood vessels and mesentery of the jejunum and ileum.

2. The difference between jejunum and ileum.

3. The shape, position and blood vessels of the vermiform appendix.

4. The surface projection of the root of the vermiform appendix (McBurney point or Lanz point) and the common sites of the vermiform appendix.

5. The features, subdivisions, blood vessels and lymphatic draining of the colon.

6. The origin, course, branches and distribution of the superior and inferior mesenteric artery.

7. The formation, relation and tributaries of the hepatic portal vein and the communications between hepatic portal and superior vena cava and inferior vena cava.

II. Comprehend

1. The structures of the inner surface of intestine.

2. The distributive feature of the artery in the intestine.

3. The concept of the mesenteric triangle.

4. The anastomoses of the colic arteries and the concept of the marginal artery.

Exercises

I. Single choice (Choose the best answer among the following four answers, and write the corresponding letter in the bracket)

1. Which organ lies in the infracolic compartment? (   )

A. Transverse colon

B. Abdominal aorta

C. Kidney

D. Suprarenal gland

2. Which of the following does **not** belong to the organs of infracolic compartment? (   )

    A. Jejunum

    B. Duodenum

    C. Ileum

    D. Colon

3. Which of the following statements about jejunum is correct? (   )

    A. The proximal 3/5 of small intestine is jejunum.

    B. It commences at the duodenojejunal flexure.

    C. It belongs to the meso-peritoneal organ.

    D. It is located in the right, upper part of the infracolic compartment.

4. The structure only distributed in ileum is (   ).

    A. aggregated lymphatic follicle

    B. solitary lymphatic follicle

    C. circular fold

    D. epiploic appendices

5. The upper end of root of mesentery is located in the (   ).

    A. right of L_2 vertebra

    B. left of L_2 vertebra

    C. right of L_3 vertebra

    D. left of L_3 vertebra

6. The superior mesenteric artery arises from abdominal aorta at the level of (   ).

    A. T_{12} B. L_1 C. L_2 D. L_3

7. The union of the splenic vein and the superior mesenteric vein is behind of the (   ).

    A. duodenum

    B. head of pancreas

    C. body of pancreas

    D. neck of pancreas

8. The inferior mesenteric vein usually enters into (   ).

    A. superior mesenteric vein

    B. hepatic vein

    C. splenic vein

    D. left gastroepiploic vein

9. The referred pain of small intestine is located in (   ).

    A. the right upper part of abdomen

    B. the right lower part of abdomen

    C. the paraumbilical part

    D. the left upper part of abdomen

10. The most common position of vermiform appendix is (   ).

    A. pre-ileal position

B. retroileal position

C. retrocecal position

D. pelvic position

11. About the vermiform appendix, which statement is correct? (   )

    A. The mesoappendix is a fan-shaped peritoneal fold.

    B. The surface projection of root of vermiform appendix is situated at the McBurney's point or Lanz point.

    C. The symptoms and signs resulting from appendicitis are same in the different position of apex.

    D. The artery supplying the appendix runs along the root of mesoappendix.

12. The appendicular artery arises from (   ).

    A. middle colic artery

    B. right colic artery

    C. the trunk of superior mesenteric artery

    D. ileocolic artery

13. The cecum is in front of the (   ).

    A. lower end of ileum

    B. right ureter

    C. psoas major

    D. iliopsoas

14. The lateral space of the ascending colon is (   ).

    A. right mesenteric sinus

    B. right iliac fossa

    C. right paracolic sulcus

    D. left paracolic sulcus

15. The branches of marginal artery are **not** distributed to (   ).

    A. transverse colon

    B. sigmoid colon

    C. descending colon

    D. ileum

16. Concerning the descending colon, which statement is **incorrect**? (   )

    A. Its upper end is continuous with transverse colon.

    B. Its lower end is continuous with sigmoid colon at the level of S_3.

    C. The left mesenteric sinus is on its medial side.

    D. The left paracolic sulcus is on its lateral side.

17. The hepatic portal vein communicates with azygos vein though the (   ).

    A. left gastric vein

    B. right gastric vein

    C. left gastroepiploic vein

    D. right gastroepiploic vein

18. The most superior branch of superior mesenteric artery is (   ).

    A. superior pancreaticoduodenal artery

    B. inferior pancreaticoduodenal artery

    C. middle colic artery

    D. right colic artery

19. The transverse colon is supplied by (   ).

    A. right colic artery

    B. left colic artery

    C. middle colic artery

    D. inferior mesenteric artery

20. Which one of the following is supplied by inferior mesenteric artery? (   )

    A. Vermiform appendix

    B. Cecum

    C. Transverse colon

    D. Descending colon

Ⅱ. Double choices (Choose the two best answers among the following answers, and write the corresponding letters in the bracket)

1. Which organs are **not** supplied by the superior mesenteric artery? (   )

    A. Cecum

    B. Ascending colon

    C. Transverse colon

    D. Descending colon

    E. Sigmoid colon

2. Which arteries are given from the inferior mesenteric artery? (   )

    A. Superior rectal artery

    B. Inferior rectal artery

    C. Right colic artery

    D. Middle colic artery

    E. Left colic artery

3. About the jejunum, which statements are **not** correct? (   )

    A. Its wall is thick.

    B. Its circular folds are large and thickly set.

    C. The blood arches and fat in its mesentery are less than ileum.

    D. There are solitary lymphatic follicles and aggregated lymphatic follicles on its mucous membrane.

    E. It is located in the right, lower part of the infracolic compartment.

4. The spaces on both sides of ascending colon are(   ).

    A. left paracolic sulcus

    B. right paracolic sulcus

    C. right mesenteric sinus

    D. left mesenteric sinus

    E. retrocecal space

5. Which alimentary canals are meso-peritoneal organs? (　　)

    A. Vermiform appendix

    B. Ascending colon

    C. Transverse colon

    D. Descending colon

    E. Sigmoid colon

6. The hepatic portal vein is formed by the union of (　　).

    A. superior mesenteric vein

    B. inferior mesenteric vein

    C. splenic vein

    D. left gastric vein

    E. right gastric vein

7. Which of the following statements about the mesentery of small intestine are **incorrect**? (　　)

    A. It is formed by a double peritoneum.

    B. The upper end of its root is at left of the L_2 vertebra.

    C. The lower end of its root is front of the right sacroiliac joint.

    D. The infection in the right mesenteric sinus can spread easily into pelvic cavity.

    E. The left mesenteric sinus is enclosed entirely.

8. The rectal venous plexus communicates with internal iliac vein though (　　).

    A. superior rectal vein

    B. inferior rectal vein

    C. anal vein

    D. median sacral vein

    E. lateral sacral vein

9. The marginal artery is **not** formed by (　　).

    A. ileocolic artery

    B. right colic artery

    C. appendicular artery

    D. left colic artery

    E. superior rectal artery

10. Which of the following statements about the cecum are **incorrect**? (　　)

    A. It is the first part of the large intestine.

    B. It is located in the right iliac region.

    C. It is relatively lower in child than in adult.

       D. It is usually an intra-peritoneal organ.

       E. The ileum opens into the anterolateral wall of cecum.

Ⅲ. **Fill the blanks (Fill the most appropriate words and phrases in the blanks)**

    1. The upper end of root of mesentery is at _____ ; its lower end is in front of the _____ . There are _____ vessels in it.

    2. The lymph of jejunum, ileum and colon finally enters into cisterna chyli through _____ trunk.

    3. The sigmoid colon is continuous with the descending colon at _____ , and it becomes rectum at _____ .

    4. The vein of vermiform appendix drains into the hepatic vein via _____ vein and _____ vein.

    5. The appendicular artery arises from _____ .

    6. The surface projection of vermiform includes _____ point and _____ point.

    7. The flexures of colon include _____ and _____ .

    8. The features of colon include _____ , _____ and _____ .

Ⅳ. **Answer the questions briefly**

    1. Describe the arteries of the colon and their origin.

    2. Describe the course and tributaries of the hepatic portal vein.

    3. Describe the lymphatic drainage of the jejunum and ileum.

    4. Describe the nerve innervation of the jejunum and ileum.

    5. Describe the mesenteric triangle.

Ⅴ. **Answer the questions in detail**

    1. Please describe the surface projection, location of vermiform appendix and tips to find in abdominal cavity.

    2. Please compare the difference and similarities of jejunum with ileum in location, blood supply and their structures.

    3. Please describe the main communications between the hepatic portal vein and systemic veins.

Section 6   The Retroperitoneal Space

Outline and Objectives

Ⅰ. **Grasp**

    1. The position, relations, blood vessels and lymphatic drainage of the kidney.

    2. The concept of renal hilum, renal sinus, renal pedicle and renal capsule.

3. The shape, three parts, three constrictions, relations and blood vessels of theureters.

4. The blood vessels (abdominal aorta, inferior vena cava) in the retroperitoneal space.

II. Comprehend

1. The conception and contents of the retroperitoneal space.

2. The shape, position and blood vessels of the suprarenal glands.

3. The position and distribution of the lumbar sympathetic trunk and celiac plexus.

Exercises

I. Single choice (Choose the best answer among the following four answers, and write the corresponding letter in the bracket)

1. Which organ does **not** lie in the retroperitoneal space? (   )

A. Abdominal aorta

B. Descending colon

C. Kidney

D. Suprarenal gland

2. Which of the following statements about the retroperitoneal space is correct? (   )

A. It is between the parietal peritoneum and visceral peritoneum of the posterior abdominal wall.

B. It is continuous with transverse fascia anteriorly.

C. It communicates with the posterior mediastinum through the superior lumbar triangle superiorly.

D. It extends into the retroperitoneal space of pelvic cavity.

3. The renal sinus does **not** include (   ).

A. renal column

B. renal pelvis

C. minor renal calyces

D. major renal calyces

4. The superior pole of left kidney is at the level of (   ).

A. the superior border of T_{11}

B. the inferior border of T_{11}

C. the superior border of T_{12}

D. the inferior border of T_{12}

5. The structure medially and posteriorly to kidney is (   ).

A. abdominal aorta

B. inferior vena cava

C. lumbar sympathetic trunk

D. genitofemoral nerve

6. The vessel behind of the right ureter is (   ).

   A. right colic vessel

   B. ileocolic vessel

   C. right common iliac vessel

   D. right external iliac vessel

7. The organ in front of the right suprarenal gland is (   ).

   A. liver

   B. gallbladder

   C. the descending part of duodenum

   D. the horizontal part of duodenum

8. Which vein does **not** enter into the inferior vena cava directly? (   )

   A. Lumbar vein

   B. Renal vein

   C. Right testicular vein

   D. Ascending lumbar vein

9. The unpaired parietal branch of the abdominal aorta is (   ).

   A. inferior phrenic artery

   B. celiac trunk

   C. median sacral artery

   D. lumbar artery

10. Concerning the lumbar ganglia, which statement is correct? (   )

    A. They belong to the parasympathetic ganglia.

    B. Their number is constant.

    C. The 1st, 2nd, and 5th lumbar ganglia are at the level of their corresponding vertebra.

    D. The 3rd and 4th lumbar ganglia are somewhat lower than their corresponding vertebra.

Ⅱ. **Double choices (Choose the two best answers among the following answers, and write the corresponding letters in the bracket)**

1. Which organs are **not** located in the retroperitoneal space? (   )

   A. Kidney

   B. Abdominal aorta

   C. Spleen

   D. Hepatic portal vein

   E. Abdominal part of ureter

2. The paired visceral branches of abdominal aorta are (   ).

   A. celiac trunk

   B. gastric artery

   C. middle suprarenal artery

    D. inferior phrenic artery

    E. renal artery

3. The muscles behind of the kidney are (   ).

    A. psoas major

    B. psoas minor

    C. quadratus lumborum

    D. transversus abdominis

    E. iliacus

4. Which of the following statements about ureter are **incorrect**? (   )

    A. It lies in retroperitoneal space.

    B. It is continuous with the renal pelvis superiorly.

    C. It is divided into four parts.

    D. There are four constriction in its course.

    E. The appendicitis of retroileal position can elicit the right ureter.

5. Which of the following statements about the suprarenal gland are **wrong**? (   )

    A. It is at the level of L_1.

    B. There is diaphragm behind it.

    C. The peritoneum fully covers its anterior surface on each side.

    D. The inferior vena cava is medial to right suprarenal gland.

    E. The abdominal aorta is medial to left suprarenal gland.

Ⅲ. Fill the blanks (Fill the most appropriate words and phrases in the blanks)

1. The upper pole of right kidney is at the level of _____ ; its lower end is at the level of _____ .

2. The upper pole of left kidney is at the level of _____ ; its lower end is at the level of _____ .

3. The covering of kidney includes _____ , _____ and _____ from outside in.

4. The contents in the renal pedicle are _____ , _____ and _____ from front to back.

5. The autonomic nerves innervating kidneys arise from _____ , which is located around _____ .

6. The superior suprarenal artery arise from _____ ; the middle suprarenal artery arise from _____ ; the inferior suprarenal artery arise from _____ .

7. The inferior vena cava is formed by the union of _____ and _____ at the level of _____ .

8. The unpaired visceral branches of abdominal aorta include _____ , _____ and _____ .

9. The right suprarenal vein enters into _____ ; the left suprarenal vein enters into _____ .

10. The celiac plexus, the largest autonomic plexus, lies in front of the upper part of __
_____ , surrounding the roots of _____ and _____ .

Ⅳ. Answer the questions briefly

1. Describe the location, boundaries and main contents in the retroperitoneal space.

2. Describe the blood supply of the suprarenal glands.

3. Describe the relation of abdominal ureter.

Ⅴ. Answer the questions in detail

1. Please describe the abdominal aorta and its branches.

2. Please depict the location, relations and coverings of kidney.

Chapter 7 The Pelvis and Perineum

Section 1 Introduction

Outline and Objectives

Ⅰ. Grasp

1. The boundaries and divisions of the perineum.
2. The boundaries and divisions of the pelvis.

Ⅱ. Comprehend

The surface anatomy (surface landmarks, rhomboid area of the lumbosacral region, sacral hiatus) of the pelvis and perineum

Exercises

Ⅰ. Single choice (Choose the best answer among the following four answers, and write the corresponding letter in the bracket)

1. The pelvis consists of the following structures **except** (   ).
    A. bony pelvis
    B. pelvic wall
    C. pelvic diaphragm
    D. renal pelvis

2. Which of the following about the greater pelvis is true? (   )
    A. The greater pelvis is also called false pelvis.
    B. The greater pelvis is the inferior part of the pelvis.
    C. The greater pelvis is only formed by bones.
    D. The inferior border of greater pelvis is pelvic diaphragm.

3. Sacral cornu is an important landmark on the surface, it is formed by (   ).
    A. the median sacral crest
    B. the spinous process of the 5th sacral vertebra
    C. the lower articular process of the 5th sacral vertebra
    D. the upper end of the intermediate sacral crest

II . **Double choices (Choose the two best answers among the following five answers, and write the corresponding letters in bracket)**

    1. Which of the following do not belong to the bony pelvis? (   )

      A. Hip bone

      B. Sacrum

      C. Coccyx

      D. Femur

      E. Lumbar vertebra

    2. Which of the following do not form the boundaries of perineum? (   )

      A. Superior border of pubic symphysis

      B. Ramus of ischium

      C. Sacrotuberous ligament

      D. Inferior ramus of pubis

      E. Sacrum

III . **Fill the blanks (Fill the most appropriate words and phrases in the blanks)**

    1. A line joining theischial tuberosities divides the perineum into _____ and _____

    ____.

    2. The pelvis is divided into the _____ and _____ by terminal line.

IV . **Answer the questions briefly**

    Describe the boundary and division of the perineum.

Section 2   The Pelvis

Outline and Objectives

I . Grasp

    1. The position, shape, relation and blood vessels (arterial supply and vein drainage) of the urinary bladder.

    2. The position, relation, blood vessels and lymphatic drainage of the rectum.

    3. The shape, position, relation and ligaments of the uterus.

    4. The arterial supply of the uterus, relationship between the uterine artery and the ureter.

    5. The shape, position and blood vessels of the ovary.

    6. The position, divisions and orifices of the uterine tube.

    7. The shape, position and relation of the prostate.

    8. The internal iliac artery and its branches in the pelvis.

Ⅱ. **Comprehend**

  1. The pelvic wall and pelvic fascia.

  2. The lymphatic drainage of the urinary bladder and uterus.

  3. The position of the seminal vesicle, ductus deferens and ejaculatory duct.

  3. The position of the pelvic venous plexuses.

Exercises

Ⅰ. **Single choice (Choose the best answer among the following four answers, and write the corresponding letter in the bracket)**

  1. The bony pelvis ( ).

   A. is formed by hip bones, sacrum, coccyx and their joints

   B. can be divided into abdominal and pelvic part by the terminal line

   C. is enclosed at the superior pelvic aperture by perineum

   D. is wider, shorter in male than in female

  2. On the lateral wall of pelvis, greater sciatic foramen is formed by ( ).

   A. lesser sciatic notch and sacrotuberous ligament

   B. greater sciatic notch and sacrospinous ligament

   C. lesser sciatic notch, sacrotuberous and sacrospinous ligaments

   D. greater sciatic notch, sacrotuberous and sacrospinous ligaments

  3. About the obturator foramen, which description is correct? ( )

   A. It is enclosed by obturator membrane completely.

   B. It is posterior to the greater sciatic foramen.

   C. Obturator canal passes through it.

   D. Obturator internus is outside the foramen.

  4. About the pelvic diaphragm, which description is correct? ( )

   A. It is formed by bones and muscles.

   B. It separates the pelvis from the perineum.

   C. The muscles in it are levator ani and sphincter ani internus.

   D. The anterior part of pelvic diaphragm is called urogenital diaphragm.

  5. About the blood vessels in the pelvis, which description is correct? ( )

   A. Common iliac artery bifurcates in front of the 4th lumbar vertebra.

   B. Common iliac vein lies anterior to the common iliac artery.

   C. External iliac vein lies medial to the external iliac artery.

   D. External iliac artery gives off the superficial epigastric artery.

  6. Which of the following is **not** a branch of anterior trunk of internal iliac artery? ( )

   A. Obturator artery

   B. Inferior gluteal artery

   C. Uterine artery

   D. Superior gluteal artery

7. Which of the following is a branch of internal iliac artery? (   )
   A. Lateral sacral artery
   B. Median sacral artery
   C. Superior rectal artery
   D. Ovarian artery

8. Which of the following is **not** formed by visceral pelvic fascia? (   )
   A. Prostate capsule
   B. Cardinal ligament of uterus
   C. Rectovesical septum
   D. Rectouterine pouch

9. Below the dentate line, the anal canal is innervated by (   ).
   A. sciatic nerve
   B. lumbar splanchnic nerve
   C. pelvic splanchnic nerve
   D. anal nerve

10. About the urinary bladder, which of the following is **not** correct? (   )
    A. Its apex is situated anteriorly and fundus posteroinferiorly.
    B. The neck of bladder is between the apex and body.
    C. When empty, it lies wholly in the lesser pelvis.
    D. When it is distended, it may raise beyond the pubic symphysis.

11. The trigone of bladder is located on (   ).
    A. fundus of bladder
    B. body of bladder
    C. apex of bladder
    D. neck of bladder

12. About the blood vessels of the bladder, which of the following is correct? (   )
    A. Superior vesical artery supplies superior part of the bladder.
    B. Inferior vesical artery supplies middle part of the bladder.
    C. Superior vesical artery also supplies the seminal vesicle.
    D. Inferior vesical artery also supplies the urogenital diaphragm.

13. About the rectum, which of the following is correct? (   )
    A. The superior part is ampulla of rectum.
    B. It begins at the level of promontory of sacrum.
    C. The sacral flexure of rectum convex forward.
    D. The perineal flexure of rectum convex forward.

14. Which of the following can be seen in the ampulla of rectum? (   )
    A. Anal column
    B. Transverse fold
    C. Anal pecten
    D. Dentate line

15. About the rectum, which of the following is correct? (   )

    A. The posterior wall is covered by peritoneum.

    B. The superior part of anterior wall is covered by peritoneum.

    C. The middle part of anterior wall is covered by peritoneum.

    D. The inferior part of anterior wall is covered by peritoneum.

16. About the artery of rectum, which of following is **not** correct? (   )

    A. The superior rectal artery is a branch of inferior mesenteric artery.

    B. The superior rectal artery divides into anterior and posterior branches.

    C. The inferior rectal artery is a branch of internal iliac artery.

    D. The inferior-superior rectal artery supplies the lower part of rectum.

17. About the prostate, which of the following is correct? (   )

    A. Its base rests on the urogenital diaphragm.

    B. The anterior part is called apex.

    C. It can be divided into 3 lobes.

    D. The part between the apex and base is the body.

18. In prostatic hypertrophy, which lobe elongates and obstructs the urethra? (   )

    A. Anterior lobe

    B. Middle lobe

    C. Posterior lobe

    D. Lateral lobe

19. About the uterus, which of the following is **not** correct? (   )

    A. It is inverted pear-shaped.

    B. The neck can be divided into supravaginal and vaginal parts.

    C. The fundus is the part below the uterine tube.

    D. Between the fundus and neck is the body of uterus.

20. About the position of uterus, which of the following is **not** correct? (   )

    A. It is situated between the urinary bladder and rectum.

    B. The position is changeable depending on the situations.

    C. Anteversion means uterus is bent forward between the body and neck.

    D. The neck is above the plane of the ischial spine.

21. Which of the following ligaments prevents the prolapse of the uterus? (   )

    A. Broad ligament

    B. Round ligament

    C. Cardinal ligament

    D. Uterosacral ligament

22. About the uterine artery, which of the following is **not** correct? (   )

    A. It arises from the internal iliac artery.

    B. It descends in front of the ureter.

    C. It gives off branches to bladder.

    D. It anastomoses with the ovarian artery.

23. About the lymphatic drainage of uterus, which of the following is **not** correct? (   )

    A. The lymph from the fundus drains to the lumbar lymph nodes.

    B. The lymph from the horn of uterus drains to the superficial inguinal lymph nodes.

    C. The lymph from the upper part of body drains to the deep inguinal lymph nodes.

    D. The lymph from the lower part of body drains to the internal iliac lymph nodes.

24. About the ovary, which of the following is **not** correct? (   )

    A. It has superior and inferior extremities.

    B. The superior extremity is embraced by the uterine tube.

    C. The proper ligament of ovary connects the inferior extremity to the uterus.

    D. The anterior border is the free border.

25. About the uterine tube, which of the following is **not** correct? (   )

    A. It occupies the free edge of the broad ligament.

    B. Each tube has 4 parts.

    C. Each tube has 2 openings.

    D. Ovarian fimbria attaches to the uterus.

26. About the ovary, which of the following is correct? (   )

    A. It is situated in the ovary fossa between the common and internal iliac arteries.

    B. It is a retroperitoneal viscera.

    C. It is connected to the uterus by proper ligament of ovary at superior extremity.

    D. It is suspended to the pelvic wall by suspensory ligament of ovary.

Ⅱ. **Double choices (Choose the two best answers among the following answers, and write the corresponding letters in the bracket)**

1. On the surface of the obturator internus, which of the following are **not** formed by the parietal pelvic fascia? (   )

    A. Obturator membrane

    B. Obturator fascia

    C. Obturator canal

    D. Tendinous arch of levator ani

    E. Pudendal canal

2. Pelvic fascial spaces include (   ).

    A. deep perineal space

    B. superficial perineal space

    C. retropubic space

    D. retrorectal space

    E. ischioanal fossa

3. Peritoneum in pelvis forms (   ).

    A. uterosacral ligament

    B. rectouterine pouch

C. round ligament of uterus

D. rectovesical septum

E. vesicouterine pouch

4. The muscles of pelvic diaphragm include (   ).

A. coccygeus

B. levator ani

C. sphincter ani internus

D. sphincter ani externus

E. piriformis

5. About pelvic part of ureter, which of the following are correct? (   )

A. It descends behind the internal iliac artery.

B. It is crossed anteriorly by the ductus deferens in male.

C. It is crossed anteriorly by the uterine artery in female.

D. Its opening is on the body of the bladder.

E. It is supplied by inferior rectal artery.

6. The arteries of rectum come from (   ).

A. superior mesenteric artery

B. femoral artery

C. superior rectal artery

D. inferior rectal artery

E. anal artery

7. Through the anterior wall of the rectum, we can **not** palpate (   ).

A. prostate

B. seminal vesicle

C. ovary

D. neck of uterus

E. urethra

8. About the relationship of the rectum, which of the following are **wrong**? (   )

A. The sacral plexus is behind it.

B. It is separated from the prostate by rectovesicalpouch in male.

C. The superior rectal artery and vein are in front of it.

D. It is separated from uterus by rectouterine pouch in female.

E. It is separated from the vagina by rectouterine pouch and fascial septum in female.

9. About the uterus, which of the following are **wrong**? (   )

A. It can be divided into four parts: apex, neck, body and fundus.

B. The isthmus is a slight constriction at the junction between the neck and body.

C. The lower part of the neck can insert into the vagina.

D. The cavity in the uterus is called uterinecanal.

E. The body is bent forward at the junction with the neck (anteflexion).

10. About the prostate, which of the following are **wrong**? (   )

    A. It is a chestnut-shaped organ.

    B. It may be divided into anterior, middle, posterior and two lateral lobes.

    C. The urethra passes through the middle lobe of the gland.

    D. There is prostatic sulcus along the middle line on the posterior surface.

    E. The ejaculatory duct penetrates the anterior lobe and opens on seminal colliculus.

11. About the vagina, which of the following are **not** correct? (   )

    A. The lower part of neck of uterus projects into it.

    B. Between neck of uterus and vaginal walls is fornix of vagina.

    C. Fornix of vagina can be divided into 2 parts: anterior part and posterior part.

    D. The anterior part of fornix of vagina is the deepest one.

    E. The lower end of vagina opens into the vaginal vestibule.

Ⅲ. Fill the blanks (Fill the most appropriate words and phrases in the blanks)

1. The parietal pelvic fascia covers anterior, posterior and lateral walls of pelvis as well as _____ and _____ (muscles).

2. On the lateral wall of pelvis, there are two ligaments, _____ and _____.

3. Obturator vessels and nerve leave the pelvis through _____.

4. The abdominal aorta bifurcates into right and left common iliac arteries in front of the _____; in front of the sacroiliac joint, common iliac artery bifurcates into _____ and _____.

5. In pelvis, the external iliac artery gives off _____ and _____.

6. The internal iliac artery gives off anterior and posteriortrunks. The parietal branches of the anterior trunk are _____ and _____.

7. The pelvic sympathetic trunks descend in front of the pelvic surface of the sacrum and unite on the coccyx to form _____. There are _____ sacral ganglia on each trunk.

8. The trigone of bladder is on the interior of the fundus. The two lateral angles are _____, the lower angle is _____.

9. The anal artery is a branch of _____, supplying the part of anal canal below _____.

10. The lymphatic vessels of the rectum drain into _____, _____ and _____.

11. _____ and _____ nerves innervate the rectum, _____ nerve innervates the anal canal below the dentate line.

12. The uterus is situated between the urinary bladder and rectum. It is bent forward between the body and neck, that is _____.

13. The neck of uterus can be divided into _____ and _____ two parts.

14. The uterine tube has 4 parts, they are _____, _____, _____ and _____.

15. The anterior border of ovary is connected to _____ , through which the ovarian vessels and nerves pass.

IV. Answer the questions briefly

1. Describe the location and division of the uterine tube.
2. Describe the lymph drainage of the rectum.
3. Describe the division and structures formed by pelvic fascia.
4. Describe the location and shape of urinary bladder.
5. Describe the main branches of the anterior trunk of internal iliac artery.
6. Describe the position and blood supply of the ovary.

V. Answer the questions in detail

1. Describe the location, relation and blood vessels of the rectum.
2. Describe the location, relation of the uterus and its support structures.

Section 3　The Perineum

Outline and Objectives

I. Grasp

1. The conception, boundaries and division of the perineum.
2. The formation and function of the pelvic diaphragm.
3. The formation and function of the urogenital diaphragm.
4. The constitution and contents of the superficial perineal space.
5. The constitution and contents of the deep perineal space.
6. The location, boundaries and main contents (branches of the pudendal nerve and internal pudendal vessels) of the ischiorectal fossa.
7. The division, curvatures and strictures of the male urethra.
8. The layers of the scrotum.
9. The structures of the spermatic cord.

II. Comprehend

1. The shape, position and function of the levator ani.
2. The blood and nerve supply of the penis and scrotum.
3. The female external genital organs.

Exercises

I . Single choice (Choose the best answer among the following four answers, and write the corresponding letter in the bracket)

1. About the perineum, which of the following is correct? (   )

    A. It is all of the soft tissue enclosing pelvic inlet.

    B. It can be divided into urogenital and anal regions.

    C. It ends anteriorly at the external reproductive organs.

    D. It ends posteriorly at the anus.

2. About the anal canal, which of the following is correct? (   )

    A. It extends from the dentate line to the anus.

    B. It is surrounded by the sphincter ani internus and externus.

    C. Sphincter aniexternus is smooth muscle.

    D. Sphincter ani externus has 2 parts: superficial and deep.

3. About the ischioanal fossa, which of the following is correct? (   )

    A. It is located between the rectum and ischium.

    B. It communicates anteriorly with the superficial perineal space.

    C. It communicates posteriorly with the gluteal region through greater sciatic foramen.

    D. The pudendal canal is located on its lateral wall.

4. Which of the following does **not** form the medial wall of the ischioanal fossa? (   )

    A. Levator ani

    B. Sphincter ani externus

    C. Superior fascia of pelvic diaphragm

    D. Inferior fascia of pelvic diaphragm

5. About the pudendal canal, which of the following is correct? (   )

    A. It runs in the center of the ischioanal fossa.

    B. It is a cleft formed by superior fascia of pelvic diaphragm.

    C. It communicates with the obturator canal.

    D. It contains the pudendal nerve and internal pudendal vessels.

6. About thepudendal nerve, which of the following is **not** correct? (   )

    A. It arises from the sacral plexus.

    B. It leaves the pelvis through the suprapiriform foramen.

    C. It gives off dorsal nerve of penis in male.

    D. It passes through the pudendal canal.

7. About the internal pudendal artery, which of the following is correct? (   )

    A. It arises from the anterior trunk of the internal iliac artery.

    B. It runs along the lateral surface of the obturator internus.

    C. It gives off the dorsal and ventral arteries of penis.

    D. It gives off perineal artery.

8. The venous blood of the anal canal drains into (   ).

   A. inferior rectal vein

   B. anal vein

   C. internal iliac vein

   D. external iliac vein

9. The lymphatic vessels from the skin of anal region drain into (   ).

   A. superficial inguinal lymph nodes

   B. deep inguinal lymph nodes

   C. internal iliac lymph nodes

   D. external inguinal lymph nodes

10. In the urogenital region, the superficial fascia of perineum is (   ).

    A. fat layer of superficial fascia

    B. superficial layer of superficial fascia

    C. deep layer of superficial fascia

    D. deep fascia

11. The superficial fascia of perineum does **not** continue with (   ).

    A. Camper's fascia of the abdominal wall

    B. Scarpa's fascia of the abdominal wall

    C. dartos coat of the scrotum

    D. superficial fascia of the penis

12. The superficial perineal space is located between (   ).

    A. skin and superficial fascia

    B. Colles' fascia and Superficial layer of superficial fascia

    C. Colles' fascia and inferior fascia of urogenital diaphragm

    D. superior fascia and inferior fascia of urogenital diaphragm

13. Which of the following is **not** in the superficial perineal space in male? (   )

    A. Superficial transverse muscle of the perineum

    B. Deep transverse muscle of the perineum

    C. Crura of penis

    D. Bulbocavernosus

14. Which of the following is **not** in the deep perineal space in male? (   )

    A. Membranous part of urethra

    B. Deep transverse muscle of perineum

    C. Bulbourethral gland

    D. Bulbocavernosus

15. The urogenital diaphragm is **not** formed by (   ).

    A. inferior fascia of urogenital diaphragm

    B. deep transverse muscle of the perineum

    C. superior fascia of urogenital diaphragm

    D. superficial fascia of perineum

16. About the perineal central tendon, which of the following is **not** correct? (   )

    A. It is also called perineal body.

    B. It lies between the anal canal and the bulb of urethra in male.

    C. It gives attachments of the levator ani.

    D. It gives attachments of the muscles of perineum.

17. The scrotum contains the following structures **except** (   ).

    A. testes

    B. epididymis

    C. lower part of the spermatic cord

    D. bulb of urethra

18. The blood of scrotum is **not** supplied by (   ).

    A. superficial external pudendal artery

    B. deep external pudendal artery

    C. superficial epigastric artery

    D. branches from internal pudendal artery

19. Which of the following nerve does **not** supply the scrotum? (   )

    A. Ilioinguinal nerve

    B. Iliohypogastric nerve

    C. Genitofemoral nerve

    D. Pudendal and posterior femoral cutaneous nerve

20. The internal spermatic fascia is derived from (   ).

    A. obliquus externus abdominus

    B. obliquus internus abdominus

    C. transverse abdominus

    D. transverse fascia

21. The distal end of the cavernous body of urethra is (   ).

    A. glans penis

    B. bulb of urethra

    C. crus penis

    D. bulbocavernosus

22. The narrowest part of the male urethra is (   ).

    A. internal orifice of urethra

    B. membranous part

    C. external orifice of urethra

    D. prostate part of urethra

23. The superficial perineal space in female contains the following **except** (   ).

    A. crura of clitoris

    B. bulbs of vestibule

    C. perineal central tendon

    D. great vestibular gland

24. Which of the following does **not** open to vaginal vestibule? (　　)

A. Vagina

B. Bulbs of vestibule

C. Female urethra

D. Great vestibular gland

25. Which of the following is **not** a structure of female external genitalorgan? (　　)

A. Mons pubis

B. Greater lips of pudendum

C. Vagina

D. Clitoris

Ⅱ. Double choices (Choose the two best answers among the following answers, and write the corresponding letters in the bracket)

1. About the ischioanal fossa, which of the following are correct? (　　)

A. Its apex lies inferiorly.

B. Its base is the perineal skin.

C. There is no fat inside the fossa.

D. It is also called ischiorectal fossa.

E. It is traversed by the obturator nerve.

2. The lateral wall of the ischioanal fossa is formed by the following **except** (　　).

A. levator ani

B. sphincter ani externus

C. ischial tuberosity

D. sacrotuberous ligament

E. fascia of obturator internus

3. About the superficial fascia of perineum, which of the following are **not** correct?
(　　)

A. It is also called Colles' fascia.

B. It is continuous with Camper's fascia.

C. It is continuous with dartos coat.

D. It is continuous with albuginea of the penis.

E. It is continuous with Scarpa's fascia.

4. The deep perineal space in female contains (　　).

A. clitoris

B. bulb of vestibule

C. great vestibular gland

D. deep transverse perineal muscle

E. urethrovaginal sphincter

5. The superficial perineal space in male does **not** contain (   ).

   A. superficial transverse muscle of peritoneum

   B. bulbourethral gland

   C. bulbocavernosus

   D. bulb of urethra

   E. deeptransverse muscle of peritoneum

6. The scrotum does **not** consist of (   ).

   A. skin.

   B. dartos coat

   C. cremaster

   D. inferior fascia of urogenital diaphragm

   E. superior fascia of urogenital diaphragm

7. The cremaster is continuous with (   ).

   A. obliquus externus abdominus

   B. obliquus internus abdominus

   C. transverse abdominus

   D. rectus abdominus

   E. dartos coat

8. About the penis, which of the following are correct? (   )

   A. It is composed of one cavernous body of penis and 2 cavernous bodies of urethra.

   B. The skin over the glans forms the prepuce.

   C. The superficial dorsal vein of penis drains into the internal pudendal vein.

   D. The superficial nerves of the penis run along the dorsum of the penis.

   E. Dorsal arteries of penis are terminal branches of the internal pudendal artery.

9. Which of the following can **not** be seen in the prostatic part of male urethra? (   )

   A. Urethral crest

   B. Seminal colliculus

   C. Prostatic sinuses

   D. Navicular fossa

   E. Opening of the bulbourethral gland

10. About the urogenital region in female, which of the following are correct? (   )

   A. Colles' fascia is the superficial fascia of perineum.

   B. The perineal central tendon in female is more elastic than that in male.

   C. The vagina does not pass through the deep perineal space.

   D. The bulbs of vestibule are located deep to the urogenital diaphragm.

   E. The greater vestibular glands are located in the deep perineal space.

Ⅲ. Fill the blanks (Fill the most appropriate words and phrases in the blanks)

1. The superficial fascia of the urogenital triangle can be divided into two layers, they are a _____ layer superficial and a _____ layer deep.

2. The sphincter ani externus has three parts, they are _____ , _____ and _____ .

3. The urogenital diaphragm is formed basically by _____ , _____ and _____ .

Ⅳ. Answer the questions briefly

1. Describe the urogenital diaphragm.
2. Describe the contents of deep perineal space.
3. Describe the wall of the scrotum.
4. Describe the anal sphincters.
5. Describe the formation of spermatic cord.

Ⅴ. Answer the questions in detail

1. Describe the formation and contents of superficial perineal space.
2. Describe the location, boundaries and contents of ischioanal fossa.
3. Describe the divisions of the male urethra.

Chapter 8 The Back and Vertebral Region

Section 1 Introduction

Outline and Objectives

Ⅰ. Grasp

1. The constitution, surface landmarks of the back and vertebral region.

2. The conception of the thoracolumbar fascia.

3. The layers of the muscles of back.

Ⅱ. Comprehend

1. The principal cutaneous nerves of the back.

2. The triangles of the back.

Exercises

Ⅰ. Single choice (Choose the best answer among the following four answers, and write the corresponding letter in the bracket)

1. Which of the following is true? (   )

    A. The sacral hiatus is the superior orifice of the sacral canal.

    B. The coccyx is a roughly triangular structure and can be palpated anterior to the a-pex of sacrum.

    C. The twelfth rib can be palpated in the lateral side of erector spinae.

    D. The spine of scapula is vertical bony crest on the scapular.

2. About the spinous process, which of the following is correct? (   )

    A. Most spinous processes cannot be palpated.

    B. The spine of the 12th is longer than others.

    C. The spines of thoracic vertebrae are long and downward sloping.

    D. The sacral spines are 7 in number.

Ⅱ. Answer the questions briefly

The boundaries and division of the back and vertebral region.

Section 2   The Layers and Structures

Ⅰ. **Single choice (Choose the best answer among the following four answers, and write the corresponding letter in the bracket)**

1. About the cutaneous nerves, which of the following is **not** right? (   )

   A. The greater occipital nerve is the branch of the anterior rami of the 2nd cervical nerve.

   B. The 3rd occipital nerve is a branch of the ramus of C3.

   C. The superior clunial nerves are the cutaneous branch of the dorsal rami of the upper three lumbar nerves.

   D. The superior gluteal cutaneous nerves supply the skin of the gluteal region.

2. Which of the following is **wrong**? (   )

   A. The nuchal fascia is situated below the trapezius.

   B. The thoracolumbar fascia covers the deep muscles of the back of the trunk.

   C. The thoracolumbar fascia passes the serratus and is continuous with the deep cervical fascia.

   D. The posterior layer of thoracolumbar fascia covers the quadratus lumborum.

3. About the muscle of the back, which of the following is **wrong**? (   )

   A. The latissimus dorsi originates from the spines of the lower six thoracic vertebrae and lumbar vertebrae.

   B. The trapezius extends from the superior nuchal line, the external occipital protuberance and the nuchal ligament.

   C. The erector spinae fills up the vertebral groove on each side of vertebral column.

   D. The erector spinae is a single muscle of back.

4. About the triangles of the back, which of the following is **wrong**? (   )

   A. The superior lumbar triangle is crossed by the subcostal, iliohypogastric and ilioinguinal nerves.

   B. The inferior lumbar triangle's floor is the obliquus internus abdominis.

   C. The suboccipital triangle is crossed by the greater occipital nerve.

   D. The superior lumbar triangle is particularly suited for auscultation.

5. The occipital artery (   ).

   A. arises from the internal carotid artery

   B. runs posterosuperiorly deep to the anterior belly of digastric

   C. anastomoses with the deep cervical artery from the subclavian artery

   D. arises from the transverse cervical artery

6. The vertebral artery (   ).

  A. arises from the carotid artery

  B. ascends through the transverse foramina of the upper 7 cervical vertebrae

  C. enters the cranial cavity through the foramen magnum

  D. joins the circle of Willis

Ⅱ. **Double choices (Choose the two best answers among the following answers, and write the corresponding letters in the bracket)**

1. Which of the following belong to the muscles of the back? (   )

  A. Latissimus dorsi

  B. Trapezius

  C. Digastric

  D. Platysma

  E. Stylohyoid

2. About the vertebral artery, which ones are right? (   )

  A. It enters the cranial cavity through the foramen magnum.

  B. It joins the circle of Willis.

  C. It ascends through the transverse foramina of the upper 7 cervical vertebrae.

  D. It arises from the common carotid artery.

  E. The vertebral arteries form the basilar artery.

Section 3   The Vertebral Canal and Its Contents

Ⅰ. **Single choice (Choose the best answer among the following four answers, and write the corresponding letter in the bracket)**

1. The vertebral canal (   ).

  A. is a bony and fibrous canal contains the vertebral artery

  B. formed by the 24 vertebral foramina and sacral canal

  C. does not contain the spinal cord

  D. does not contain the spinal meninges

2. About the spinal meninges, which of the following is **incorrect**? (   )

  A. The spinal dura mater is continuous with the dura of the brain.

  B. The dura mater encloses the terminal filum.

  C. The arachnoid mater is continuous with the cerebral arachnoid.

  D. The dura mater forms the denticulate ligament.

3. About the spinal space, which of the following is **incorrect**? (   )

  A. The epidural space lies between the spinal dura mater and the periosteum of the vertebrae.

  B. The subdural space does not communicate with the subarachnoid space.

C. The subarachnoid space is the interval between the arachnoid and pia mater.

D. The subdural space is full of the CSF.

4. About the subarachnoid space, which of the following is **wrong**? (   )

A. It is the interval between the arachnoid and pia mater.

B. It contains the cerebral spinal fluid.

C. It becomes narrower from the lower end of spinal cord.

D. Terminal cistern is the best site for a lumbar puncture.

II. Answer the questions briefly

Depict the subarachnoid space.

Answers

Chapter 1　The Head

Section 1　Introduction

Ⅰ. Single choice

    C

Ⅱ. Double choices

    BD

Ⅲ. Fill the blanks

    1. sphenoid bone, frontal bone, parietal bone, temporal bone

    2. cranium, face, supraorbital margin, zygomatic arch, superior margin of external a-coustic meatus, mastoid process

Ⅳ. Answer the questions briefly

    1. The head is separated from the neck by an imaginary line linking with the lower border of mandible, angle of mandible, mastoid process, superior nuchal line and the external occipital protuberance. The head is divided into cranium and face with an imaginary line linking with the supraorbital margin, zygomatic arch, superior margin of external acoustic meatus and mastoid process.

    2. The supraorbital foramen lies on the superior margin of the orbit about 2.5 cm from the median line. It transmits the supraorbital artery, vein and nerve. The infraorbital foramen locates about 0.5 - 0.8 cm below the infraorbital margin, about 2.5 cm from the median line. It transmits the infraorbital artery, vein and nerve. The mental foramen lies about 2.5 cm from the median fusion of the two halves of the mandible and halfway between the edge of the gum and the lower border of the mandible. It transmits the mental artery, vein and nerve.

Section 2　The Face

Ⅰ. Single choice

    1. C　2. D　3. A　4. D　5. C　6. A　7. D　8. C　9. C　10. D

II. Double choices

1. BD   2. BD   3. DE   4. DE   5. CE

III. Fill the blanks

1. external carotid artery, auriculotemporal nerve, retromandibular vein, superficial temporal vessels

2. facial nerve and its branches, maxillary vessels, transverse facial vessels

3. angular vein, internal jugular vein

4. temporal branch, zygomatic branch, buccal branch, marginal mandibular branch, cervical branch

5. inferior alveolar artery, middle meningeal artery

IV. Answer the questions briefly

1. The structures passing through the parotid gland vertically are external carotid artery, auriculotemporal nerve, retromandibular vein and superficial temporal vessels.

2. The structures passing through the parotid gland transversely are facial nerve and its branches, maxillary vessels, and transverse facial vessels.

3. Parotid duct begins from the anterior border of the superficial part of the gland, passes forwards about 1 cm below the zygomatic arch, crosses the surface of the masseter, and then turns medially through the buccinator, and lastly opens to the mucous membrane opposite to the second upper molar tooth. The buccal branch of the facial nerve and the transverse facial vessels run accompanying with the parotid duct.

4. The mandibular nerve has two trunks, anterior and posterior. The branches of anterior trunk are those innervating the masticatory muscles and the buccal nerve. The branches of posterior trunk are the auriculotemporal nerve, lingual nerve and the inferior alveolar nerve.

5. The masticatory muscles contain the temporalis, masseter, medial pterygoid and lateral pterygoid. They are innervated by the posterior trunk of the mandibular nerve.

V. Answer the questions in detail

1. The structures passing through the parotid gland are the external carotid artery, auriculotemporal nerve, retromandibular vein, superficial temporal vessels, facial nerve and its branches, maxillary vessels and transverse facial vessels. Among them, the external carotid artery, auriculotemporal nerve, retromandibular vein and superficial temporal vessels run through the gland vertically, and the facial nerve and its branches, maxillary vessels and transverse facial vessels run through the gland transversely.

From superficial to deep, these structures are arranged in facial nerve and its branches, retromandibular vein, external carotid artery and auriculotemporal nerve.

2. The maxillary artery can be divided into 3 parts. The first part lies between the neck of mandible and the lower margin of lateral pterygoid. The chief branches of this part are the inferior alveolar artery and middle meningeal artery. The second part runs superficially or

deeply to the lateral pterygoid. It gives the buccal artery and the arteries for masticatory muscles. The third part lies between the upper margin of lateral pterygoid and the pterygo-palatine fossa. Its chief branches are the posterior superior alveolar artery and infraorbital artery.

Section 3   The Cranium

I. Single choice

1. D   2. C   3. D   4. B   5. B   6. D   7. C   8. B   9. D   10. C

II. Double choices

1. AE   2. CD   3. AE   4. AB   5. AB

III. Fill the blanks

1. skin, superficial fascia, epicranial aponeurosis

2. skin, superficial fascia, temporal fascia, temporalis, pericranium

3. skin, superficial fascia, epicranial aponeurosis, subaponeurotic loose connective tissue, pericranium

4. oculomotor nerve, trochlear nerve, ophthalmic nerve, maxillary nerve

5. internal carotid artery, abducent nerve

IV. Answer the questions briefly

1. There are five layers of the front-oparieto-occipital region. From superficial to deep, they are skin, superficial fascia, epicranial aponeurosis, subaponeurotic loose connective tissue and pericranium.

2. There are five layers of the temporal region. From superficial to deep, they are skin, superficial fascia, temporal fascia, temporalis and pericranium.

3. The cavernous sinus lies on each side of the sella turcica and extends from the superior orbital fissure to the apex of the petrous part of temporal bone. The internal carotid artery and abducent nerve pass through the medial wall of the cavernous sinus. The oculomotor nerve, trochlear nerve, ophthalmic nerve, maxillary nerve pass through the lateral wall of the cavernous sinus.

4. The cerebral dura mater projects into the cranial cavity to form the cerebral falx, tentorium of cerebellum, cerebellar falx and diaphragm sella. In some places, two layers of cerebral dura mater separate to form the venous sinuses. They are the superior sagittalsinus, inferior sagittal sinus, straight sinus, confluence of sinus, transverse sinus, sigmoid sinus and cavernous sinus.

V. Answer the questions in detail

Layers: There are five layers of the front-oparieto-occipital region. From superficial to deep, they are skin, superficial fascia, epicranial aponeurosis, subaponeurotic loose connective tissue and pericranium.

Characteristics: ①The skin is thick and dense, consists of abundant blood supply, hair bulbs, sweat glands and sebaceous glands. ② The superficial fascia is divided into many 'pockets' by the dense connective tissue. Therefore, the inflammation can be limited in this layer. There is a lot of bleeding after trauma because the wall of vessels could not contract by adherence with the fibrous bands. ③Epicranial aponeurosis is tough and dense. It connects the frontal belly and occipital belly of occipitofrontalis and is continuous with the temporal fascia laterally. ④Subaponeurotic loose connective tissue is the loose connective tissue which is located between the scalp proper and the pericranium. Blood, pus and infection may spread in this space during trauma or inflammation ⑤Pericranium is thin and dense. It closely adheres to the sutures of cranial bones. Therefore, the subpericranial hematoma usually limits within a piece of cranial bone.

Chapter 2   The Neck

Section 1   Introduction

Ⅰ. Single choice

1. A   2. C   3. C   4. B   5. D   6. A   7. A   8. B   9. C   10. A

Ⅱ. Double choices

1. AD   2. CE   3. BC   4. BD   5. AD

Ⅲ. Fill the blanks

1. anterior region, lateral region, sternocleidomastoid region

2. submental triangle, submandibular triangle

3. carotid triangle, muscular triangle

4. anterior margin of sternocleidomastoid, posterior belly of digastric, superior belly of omohyoid

5. posterior margin of sternocleidomastoid, anterior margin of trapezius, inferior belly of omohyoid

Ⅳ. Answer the questions briefly

1. The boundaries of the muscular triangle are the anterior margin of sternocleidomastoid, the superior belly of omohyoid and the median line of the neck.

2. The boundaries of the carotid triangle are the anterior margin of sternocleidomastoid, the posterior belly of digastric and the superior belly of omohyoid.

3. The boundaries of thesubmandibular triangle are the lower border of the mandible and the two bellies of digastric.

Ⅴ. Answer the questions in detail

The neck is bounded superiorly by an imaginary line linking with the lower border of mandible, angle of mandible, mastoid process, superior nuchal line and the external occipital protuberance; inferiorly by the upper border of sternum, the clavicle and a line extending from the acromion to the spine of the 7th cervical vertebra.

The neck can be divided into two portions by the anterior margin of the trapezius. The posterior portion is nape, and the anterior portion is the side of neck. The side of neck is subdivided by the sternocleidomastoid into three regions, the anterior region, the lateral region and the sternocleidomastoid region.

The anterior region of the neck is subdivided by hyoid bone into suprahyoid and infrahyoid regions. The suprahyoid region consists of submental triangle and submandibular triangle. The infrahyoid region consists of carotid triangle and muscular triangles.

The lateral region contains occipital triangle and supraclavicular fossa.

Section 2   The Superficial Structures and Cervical Fascia

Ⅰ. Single choice

1. B   2. C   3. B   4. B   5. A   6. B   7. B   8. C   9. D   10. C   11. B   12. B   13. C
14. C   15. D

Ⅱ. Double choices

1. BE   2. BD   3. AC   4. CD   5. BE

Ⅲ. Fill the blanks

1. sternocleidomastoid, trapezius, parotid gland, submandibular gland

2. investing fascia, visceral fascia, prevertebral fascia

3. posterior division of retromandibular vein, posterior auricular vein, subclavian vein

4. axillary artery, axillary vein, brachial plexus

5. common carotid artery, internal carotid artery, internal jugular vein, vagus nerve

Ⅳ. Answer the questions briefly

1. The enveloping fascia is attached posteriorly to the nuchal ligament and the spine of the 7th cervical vertebra, superiorly to the lower border of mandible, zygomatic arch, mastoid process, superior nuchal line and the external occipital protuberance, inferiorly to the jugular notch, clavicle and the acromion. It divides into two layers to enclose two muscles (sternocleidomastoid, trapezius) and two glands (submandibular and parotid glands) to form their sheath.

2. The prevertebral fascia extends from the base of skull to the third thoracic vertebra, where it fuses with the anterior longitudinal ligament. Laterally, it surrounds the axillary artery, axillary vein, and brachial plexus to form their sheath, the axillary sheath.

3. The carotid sheath is formed by the cervical fascia and extends from the base of skull

to the root of neck. It encloses the common carotid artery, internal carotid artery, internal jugular vein and the vagus nerve.

4. Above the upper border of manubrium sterni, the enveloping fascia divides into two layers to attach to its anterior and posterior margins, to form the suprasternal space. The sternal head of sternocleidomastoid, anterior jugular vein, jugular venous arch, lymph nodes and fatty tissue are in this space.

5. The pretracheal space is a potential space in front of the trachea and behind the infrahyoid muscles and pretracheal fascia. The pretracheal lymph nodes, inferior thyroid vein, unpaired thyroid venous plexus, the lowest thyroid artery, brachiocephalic trunk and left brachiocephalic vein are in this space. In children, the upper part of thymus is also in this space.

V. Answer the questions in detail

1. The cervical fascia has three layers. From superficial to deep, they are enveloping fascia, pretracheal fascia and prevertebral fascia.

The enveloping fascia is attached posteriorly to the nuchal ligament and the spine of the 7th cervical vertebra, superiorly to the lower border of mandible, zygomatic arch, mastoid process, superior nuchal line and the external occipital protuberance, inferiorlyto the jugular notch, clavicle and the acromion. It forms the sheath for two muscles (sternocleidomastoid, trapezius) and two glands (submandibular and parotid glands).

The pretracheal fascia extends from the hyoid, thyroid cartilage and the arch of the cricoid cartilage, downward into the thorax and blends laterally connecting with the carotid sheath. It forms the thyroid sheath and the suspensory ligament of thyroid gland.

The prevertebral fascia extends from the base of skull to the third thoracic vertebra, where it fuses with the anterior longitudinal ligament. Laterally, it surrounds the axillary artery, axillary vein, and brachial plexus to form their sheath, the axillary sheath.

2. The superficial nerves of the neck contain the branches of the facial nerve and the cutaneous branches of the cervical plexus.

The branches of the facial nerve in neck are the marginal mandibular branch and cervical branch. The marginal mandibular branch supplies the muscles of the lower lip and chin. The cervical branch supplies the platysma.

There are 4 cutaneous branches of the cervical plexus. They appear at the midpoint of the posterior border of the sternocleidomastoid. The lesser occipital nerve is distributed to the skin and scalp behind the ear. The greater auricular nerve supplies much of the external ear and some skin of the face below and in front of the ear. The transverse nerve of neck supplies most of the skin of the anterior part of neck. The supraclavicular nerve supplies the skin of the anterolateral neck, upper thorax and shoulder.

Section 3   The Anterior Region of the Neck

I. Single choice

1. D   2. C   3. B   4. C   5. D   6. B   7. C   8. D   9. D   10. D   11. C   12. C   13. B 14. D   15. C

II. Double choices

1. DE   2. BE   3. AC   4. BC   5. AB

III. Fill the blanks

1. suprahyoid region, infrahyoid region

2. anterior margin of sternocleidomastoid, posterior belly of digastric, superior belly of omohyoid

3. sternohyoid, omohyoid, sternothyroid, thyrohyoid

4. enveloping fascia, pretracheal fascia

5. external carotid artery, thyrocervical trunk

6. aortic arch, subclavian artery

IV. Answer the questions briefly

1. **Boundaries:** The submandibular triangle is enclosed by the lower border of mandible, two bellies of digastric. Deeply, there are mylohyoid and hyoglossus; superficially, it is covered by the skin, superficial fascia, platysma and the enveloping fascia.

    Contents: It contains the submandibular gland, submandibular lymph nodes, facial artery and vein, lingual artery and vein, lingual nerve and hypoglossal nerve.

2. **Boundaries:** The carotid triangle is enclosed by the anterior margin of sternocleidomastoid, posterior belly of digastric and the superior belly of omohyoid. Deeply, there is prevertebral fascia; superficially, it is covered by the skin, superficial fascia, platysma and the enveloping fascia.

    Contents: It contains the internal jugular vein and its tributaries, common carotid artery and its branches, hypoglossal nerve and its descending branch, vagus nerve and its branches, and some lymph nodes.

3. **Boundaries:** The muscular triangle is enclosed by the anterior margin of sternocleidomastoid, superior belly of omohyoid and the median line of neck. Deeply, there is prevertebral fascia; superficially, it is covered by the skin, superficial fascia, platysma, superficial veins, cutaneous nerves and the enveloping fascia.

    Contents: It contains the sternohyoid, sternothyroid, thyrohyoid, superior belly of omohyoid, pretracheal fascia, thyroid gland, parathyroid gland and cervical parts of esophagus and trachea.

4. The cervical part of trachea is covered from outer inwards by the skin, superficial fascia, enveloping fascia, suprasternal space, infrahyoid muscles and the pretracheal fascia. The

isthmus of thyroid gland usually lies over the 2nd, 3rd and 4th tracheal rings. Below the isthmus, there are the inferior thyroid vein, unpaired thyroid jugular arch and the lowest thyroid artery.

V. Answer the questions in detail

1. **Location:** The thyroid consists of two lateral lobes and one isthmus. The isthmus extends across the 2nd, 3rd and 4th tracheal rings. The lateral lobes overlap the sides of the larynx and trachea, and extend from the oblique line of thyroid gland to the 5th or 6th tracheal ring.

Relationship: Anterior (from outside inwards): the skin, the superficial fascia, the enveloping fascia, the infrahyoid muscles and the pretracheal fascia. Posteromedial aspect of each lobe: the larynx and trachea, the pharynx and esophagus, and the recurrent laryngeal nerve. Lateral to each lobe: the carotid sheath and the sympathetic trunk.

Coverings: It is enclosed by two coverings. The outer covering is a sheath of the pretracheal fascia (the thyroid sheath, false capsule); and the inner covering is its own fibrous capsule (the true capsule).

2. **Arteries:** ① Superior thyroid artery: It arises from the external carotid artery and distributes to the superior pole of the gland. It accompanies firstly with the superior laryngeal nerve and its external laryngeal nerve, and then leaves the nerve about 1 cm above the superior pole of the gland. ②Inferior thyroid artery: It arises from the thyrocervical trunk of the subclavian artery and accompanies with the recurrent laryngeal nerve. Near the lower pole of gland, recurrent laryngeal nerve crosses in front of or behind the artery. ③Lowest thyroid artery: It is occasional unpaired artery arising from the aortic arch or the brachiocephalic trunk. It ascends in front of the trachea to reach the isthmus of the gland.

Veins: ①The superior thyroid vein arises from the upper pole of the lateral lobe and runs upwards with the superior thyroid artery to drain into the internal jugular vein. ②The middle thyroid vein arises near the lateral border of the gland and passes across the common carotid artery to enter the internal jugular vein. ③The inferior thyroid vein arises from the network on the isthmus and opens into the brachiocephalic vein in front of the trachea.

Considerations: According to the relationship between thyroid arteries and laryngeal nerves, the superior thyroid artery must be ligated and sectioned near the upper pole of the gland, the inferior thyroid artery must be ligated some distance lateral to the thyroid gland in subtotal thyroidectomy.

Section 4   The Sternocleidomastoid Region of the Neck

I. Single choice

　　1. D　　2. B　　3. A　　4. A　　5. B　　6. B　　7. A　　8. C

II. Double choices

　　1. DE　　2. BE　　3. AD　　4. BE　　5. CE

Ⅲ. Fill the blanks

1. 1st to 4th cervical nerves

2. hypoglossal nerve, anterior branches of the 2nd and 3rd cervical nerves

3. sternohyoid, omohyoid, sternothyroid

4. common carotid artery, internal carotid artery, internal jugular vein, vagus nerve

5. lesser occipital nerve, greater auricular nerve, transverse nerve of neck, supraclavicular nerve

6. aortic arch, right subclavian artery

Ⅳ. Answer the questions briefly

1. It is formed by two roots. The upper root arises from the hypoglossal nerve (Its fibers derive from the anterior branch of the first cervical nerve), and the lower root arises from the anterior branches of the 2nd and 3rd cervical nerves. The ansa sends branches to innervate the sternothyroid, sternohyoid and omohyoid.

2. Above the upper border of thyroid cartilage, the carotid sheath encloses the internal carotid artery, internal jugular vein and the vagus nerve. Below the upper border of thyroid cartilage, the carotid sheath encloses the common carotid artery, internal jugular vein and the vagus nerve.

3. Cervical plexus is formed by the anterior branches of the upper four cervical nerves. It lies under the upper half of the sternocleidomastoid and on the anterior surface of the scalenus medius. Its main branches are the lesser occipital nerve, greater auricular nerve, transverse nerve of neck, supraclavicular nerve and phrenic nerve.

Ⅴ. Answer the questions in detail

Location: It extends from the base of the skull to the root of neck where it is continuous with the mediastinum.

Relationship: Anterior to the sheath are the sternocleidomastoid, sternohyoid, sternothyroid and omohyoid. The ansa cervicalis may lie on the surface of carotid sheath. Posteriorly, the sympathetic trunk and the prevertebral muscles are located beneath the prevertebral fascia. On the medial side of sheath, there are pharynx, esophagus, larynx, trachea, recurrent laryngeal nerve and the lateral lobe of thyroid gland.

Contents: In the carotid sheath, the common and internal carotid artery lies on the medial side, the internal jugular vein lies on the lateral side, and the vagus nerve descends behind and between these vessels. The common carotid artery divides into internal and external carotid arteries at the upper border of thyroid cartilage. Therefore, above the upper border of thyroid cartilage, the carotid sheath encloses the internal carotid artery, internal jugular vein and the vagus nerve; below the upper border of thyroid cartilage, the carotid sheath encloses the common carotid artery, internal jugular vein and the vagus nerve.

Section 5   The Lateral Region of the Neck

Ⅰ. Single choice

1. A   2. D   3. C   4. B   5. B   6. A   7. C   8. C   9. D   10. A   11. C   12. C   13. C
14. A

Ⅱ. Double choices

1. AB   2. CE   3. CE   4. BE   5. BD   6. AC   7. BD   8. CD

Ⅲ. Fill the blanks

1. occipital triangle, greater supraclavicular fossa, inferior belly of omohyoid

2. subclavian artery, brachial plexus

3. aortic arch, brachiocephalic trunk, first rib

4. vertebral artery, thyrocervical trunk, internal thoracic artery, costocervical trunk

5. suprascapular nerve, dorsal scapular nerve, long thoracic nerve

6. subclavian vein, internal jugular vein, thoracic duct, right lymphatic duct

Ⅳ. Answer the questions briefly

1. The subclavian artery is divided into three parts by scalenus anterior: the first part is medial to it, and the second part is behind it, and the third part lateral to it. Main branches of this artery are the vertebral artery, thyrocervical trunk, internal thoracic artery and the costocervical trunk.

2. The occipital triangle is enclosed by the posterior border of sternocleidomastoid, anterior border of trapezius and the inferior belly of omohyoid. Its roof is enveloping fascia. The floor is formed by the levator scapula, scalenus anterior, medius and posterior. The main contents of this triangle are external branch of accessory nerve, lateral jugular lymph nodes and some cutaneous branches of cervical plexus.

3. The accessory nerve enters the lateral region under the enveloping fascia at the junction of the upper and middle thirds of the posterior border of sternocleidomastoid. The external branch of accessory nerve runs obliquely downwards across the occipital triangle to end in the trapezius at the junction of the middle and lower thirds of its anterior border. Its muscular branches innervate the sternocleidomastoid and trapezius.

4. The scalene fissure is bounded by the scalenus anterior, scalenus medius and the first rib. The subclavian artery and brachial plexus pass through this fissure.

5. The venous angle is at the junction of subclavian vein and internal jugular vein. The left venous angle receives the drainage of thoracic duct, and the right venous angle receives the drainage of right lymphatic duct.

6. The boundaries of the triangle of vertebral artery are the longus colli (medially), scalenus anterior (laterally) and the first part of the subclavian artery. In this triangle, there are mainly the vertebral artery and vein, inferior thyroid artery, cervical sympathetic trunk and

the cervicothoracic sympathetic ganglion etc.

V. Answer the questions in detail

1. **Location:** It covers the apex of the lung and extends through the thoracic inlet into the root of neck for 2. 5 cm above the middle of the clavicle.

Relationship: Anteriorly: there is subclavian artery with its branches, scalenus anterior, phrenic nerve, vagus nerve, subclavian vein and the cervical part of thoracic duct. Posteriorly, there are sympathetic trunk and the anterior branch of the first thoracic nerve. Laterally, it is related to the scalenus medius and brachial plexus. Medially, there are the subclavian artery and brachiocephalic vein on the left side and the brachiocephalic artery, brachiocephalic vein and trachea on the right side.

2. **Origin and insertion:** Scalenus anterior arises from the anterior tubercles of the transverse processes of the third to sixth cervical vertebrae, and its fibers extend downward and slightly laterally to insert on the upper edge of the first rib, in front of the subclavian groove.

Relationship: Anteriorly: There are the phrenic nerve, subclavian vein, suprascapular artery, transverse cervical artery, vagus nerve and the thoracic duct. Posteriorly, there are the subclavian artery and the brachial plexus.

Chapter 3   The upper Limb

Section 1   Introduction

I. Single choice

1. C   2. D

II. Fill the blanks

1. scapular region, pectoral region, axilla
2. cephalic vein, basilic vein, median cubital vein

Section 2   The Shoulder

I. Single choice

1. D   2. C   3. D   4. C   5. A   6. C   7. B   8. D   9. C   10. C   11. D   12. C

II. Double choices

1. AE   2. BD   3. BD   4. DE   5. BE

III. Fill the blanks

1. first rib, middle part of clavicle, superior border of scapula
2. pectoralis major, pectoralis minor, clavipectoral fascia, subclavius

3. latissimus dorsi, teres major, subscapularis, scapula

4. cephalic vein, lateral pectoral nerve, thoracoacromial vessels

5. three, pectoralis minor

6. circumflex scapular vessels; axillary nerve, posterior humeral circumflex vessels

7. lateral group, pectoral (anterior) group, subscapular (posterior) group, central group, apical group

8. superior scapular artery, dorsal scapular artery, circumflex scapular artery

9. axillary nerve

10. suprascapular, infrascapularis, teres major, subscapularis

IV. Answer the questions briefly

1. The quadrangular space is a structure of posterior wall of axilla. Its superior border is formed by the teres minor and subscapularis; the inferior border by teres major; the lateral border by the surgical neck of humerus; the medial border by the long head of triceps brachii. The structure passing through it are the axillary nerve and the posterior humeral circumflex vessels.

2. The anterior wall of axillary cavity is formed by the pectoralis major, pectoralis minor, clavipectoral fascia and subclavius. The clavipectoral fascia lies between the superior border of pectoralis minor and subclavius that is passed through by the cephalic vein, lateral pectoral nerve and thoracoacromial vessels.

3. The muscles of shoulder include the deltoid, supraspinatus, infraspinatus, teres minor, teres major and subscapularis. The tendons of the supraspinatus, infraspinatus, teres minor and subscapularis form the shoulder cuff fusing with the underlying capsule of shoulder joint and strengthen it.

4. The axillary artery is divided into three segments by the pectoralis minor overlying it anteriorly. The first segment lies superior to the upper border of pectoralis minor and gives off the superior thoracic artery. The second segment lies behind the muscle and gives off the thoracoacromial artery and the lateral thoracic artery. The third segmentlies inferior to lower border of pectoralis minor and gives off the subscapular artery, the posterior humeral circumflex artery and anterior humeral circumflex artery.

5. The axillary lymph nodes are divided into five groups collecting lymphatic vessels from thoracic wall, breast, upper back and upper limb. Lateral group is arranged along distal part of axillary vein to receive lymph of upper limb; pectoral group along lateral thoracic vessels to receive lymph of thoracic wall and breast; subscapular group along subscapular vessels to receive lymph of scapular region, posterior thoracic wall and back; central group is embedded in fat of axilla to receive the output lymphatic vessels of the above three groups; apical group are arranged along the proximal part of axillary vein, receiving the output of the four groups, and finally form the subclavian trunk.

V. Answer the questions in detail

1. The axilla lies between the upper part of arm and lateral wall of chest, beneath the shoulder joint. It is pyramidal in shape and has an apex, a bottom and four walls.

Apex: It is upward and triangle in shape surrounded by the first rib, middle part of clavicle and upper edge of scapula.

Bottom: It is downward and formed by skin, superficial fascia and axillary fascia.

Four walls: The anterior wall is formed by pectoralis major, pectoralis minor, subclavius and clavipectoral fascia that is passed through by the cephalic vein, lateral pectoral nerve and thoracoacromial vessels.

The posterior wall is formed by the latissimus dorsi, teres major, subscapularis and scapula. There is a triangular space (medially) and a quadrangular space (laterally) on it divided by the long head of triceps brachii. Its superior border is formed by the teres minor and subscapularis; the inferior border by teres major; the lateral border by the surgical neck of humerus. The structures passing through the quadrangular are the axillary nerve and the posterior humeral circumflex vessels, the triangularis circumflex humeral vessels.

The medial wall is formed by the anterior serratus, upper 4 ribs and corresponding intercostal muscle.

The lateral wall is formed by the intertubercular sulcus of humerus, biceps brachiiand coracobrachialis.

2. The contents of axilla include axillary artery, axillary vein and brachial plexus, which are wrapped in axillary sheath together and axillary lymph nodes.

Axillary artery: It is divided into three segments by the pectoralis minor. The first segment gives off the superior thoracic artery. The second segment gives off the thoracoacromial artery and the lateral thoracic artery. The third segment gives off the subscapular, the posterior humeral circumflex and anterior humeral circumflex arteries.

The axillary vein is located in the anteromedial part of the axillary artery.

The brachial plexus encloses the axillary artery in three bundles. The lateral bundle includes the musculocutaneous nerve and the lateral root of the median nerve; the medial bundle includes the medial root of the median nerve, the ulnar nerve, the medial cutaneous nerve of the forearm and the medial cutaneous nerve of the arm; and the posterior bundle includes the axillary nerve, the radial nerve and thoracodorsal nerve. In addition, brachial plexus also has some small branches: lateral pectoral nerve, medial pectoral nerve, subscapular nerve, superior scapular nerve and long thoracic nerve.

The axillary lymph nodes are divided into five groups. Lateral lymph nodes are arranged along distal part of axillary vein to receive lymph of upper limbs; pectoral lymph nodes along lateral thoracic vessels to receive lymph of chest wall and breast; subscapular lymph nodes along subscapular vessels to receive lymph of scapular region, posterior thoracic wall and back; central lymph nodes are embedded in fat of axilla to receive the output lymphatic vessels of the above three groups; apical lymph nodes are arranged along the proximal part of axillary vein, receiving the output of the four groups, and finally form the subclavian trunk.

Section 3   The Arm

Ⅰ. Single choice

1. A   2. B   3. A   4. D   5. C   6. B   7. C   8. D   9. A   10. A

Ⅱ. Double choices

1. DE   2. AD   3. BD   4. DE   5. BD

Ⅲ. Fill the blanks

1. groove for radial nerve

2. radial nerve

3. triceps brachii, groove for radial nerve

4. lateral superior brachial cutaneous nerve, inferior lateral brachial cutaneous nerve, medial brachial cutaneous nerve, costobrachial nerve

5. basilic vein, brachial artery, brachial vein, median nerve, ulnar nerve

6. radial nerve, deep brachial vessels

7. anterior muscles of arm, musculocutaneous nerve, brachial vessels, median nerve, ulnar nerve

8. deep brachial artery, nutrient artery of humerus, superior ulnar collateral artery, inferior ulnar collateral artery

9. cephalic vein, lateral antebrachial cutaneous nerve

10. triceps brachii, radial nerve, deep brachial vessels

Ⅳ. Answer the questions briefly

1. The humeromuscular tunnel is situated in the back of the middle part of the arm. It's formed by the three heads of triceps brachii and the sulcus of radial nerve. The radial nerve and deep brachial vessels pass through in it. Because the radial nerve is close to the bony surface, lesion is easy to the radial nerve when fracture happened in the middle part of the humerus and resulting in paralysis of the extensor muscle of the forearm and wrist drop.

2. There are two neurovascular bundles located in the medial and lateral grooves of biceps brachii. The lateral neurovascular bundle includes the terminal branch of musculocutaneous nerve (lateral antebrachial cutaneous nerve) and the cephalic vein. The medial neurovascular bundle contains the brachial artery and veins, the basilic vein, the median nerve, the ulnar nerve, the radial nerve, etc.

Ⅴ. Answer the questions in detail

The muscles of arm can be divided into anterior and posterior groups.

Anterior group muscles include the biceps brachii, the coracobrachialis and the brachialis, which all are innervated by the musculocutaneous nerve. The long head of biceps brachii originates from the supraglenoid tubercle while the short head originates from the coracoid process of scapula, they fuse together and inserts into the radial tuberosity. Its main function is to flex elbow joints, additionally, to make the pronate forearm supinate. The coracobrachialis begins at the coracoid process of scapula and ends into the middle part of the humerus flexing and adducting the shoulder joint. The brachialis begins in the middle part of the humerus and inserts into the ulnar tuberosity flexing the elbow joint.

The posterior group muscles are triceps brachii and anconeus, which all are supplied by the radial nerve. The long head of triceps brachii originates from the infraglenoid tubercle of scapula while the lateral and medial heads above and below the sulcus of radial nerve of humerus respectively, they fuse together and insert to olecranon. Its main action is to extend elbow joint.

Section 4　The Elbow

Ⅰ. Single choice

1. B　2. B　3. D　4. C　5. C　6. A　7. B　8. A　9. C　10. D

Ⅱ. Double choices

1. CE　2. CD　3. CE　4. BC　5. DE

Ⅲ. Fill the blanks

1. olecranon of ulna, medial epicondyle of humerus, lateral epicondyle of humerus

2. cephalic vein, basilic vein

3. lateral cubital triangle

4. elbow joint

5. pronator teres, brachioradialis

6. brachialis, capsule of elbow joint

7. tendon of biceps brachii, median, radial

8. ulnar nerve

9. radial, ulnar

10. humeroradial, humeroulnar, proximal radioulnar

Ⅳ. Answer the questions briefly

1. The arterial rete of the elbow joint is formed by the anastomoses of several arteries. Such as radial collateral artery (from deep brachial artery) with the radial recurrent artery (from radial artery), the middle collateral artery (from deep brachial artery) with the interosseous recurrent artery (from interosseous artery), and the superior and inferior ulnar collateral arteries (from the brachial artery) with the ulnar collateral artery (from ulnar artery).

2. When elbow flexion is at the right angle, the medial and lateral epicondyles of humerus and the olecranon of ulna form an isosceles triangle, which is called posterior cubital triangle. When the elbow extension is fully straight, the above three points form a straight

line. The isosceles triangle relationship can be changed because of the dislocation of elbow or the fracture of medial and lateral epicondyles of humerus. However, the fracture of other parts of the humerus will not affect the triangular or linear relationship.

V. Answer the questions in detail

The cubital fossa is triangular depression and located in front of the elbow joint.

The upper boundary is an imaginary line between the medial and lateral epicondyles of the humerus; the lower lateral boundary is the brachioradialis; the lower medial boundary is the pronator teres; the roof is composed of the skin, superficial fascia and deep fascia; the floor is composed of brachialis and supinator.

The tendon of biceps brachii is located in the center of the cubital fossa, the brachial vessels and the median nerve covered by the bicipital aponeurosis is medial to it from the lateral medially, and the radial nerve is lateral to it.

The brachial artery is divided into radial artery and ulnar artery in the middle point of cubital fossa and at the level of neck of radius. The median nerve passes through pronator teres into forearm. The radial nerve is between the brachioradialis and tendon of biceps brachii bifurcating into the superficial and deep branches.

Section 5   The Forearm

I. Single choice

1. D   2. B   3. C   4. B   5. D   6. D   7. B   8. D   9. A   10. C

II. Double choices

1. BE   2. DE   3. DE   4. BD   5. AC

III. Fill the blanks

1. cephalic vein, basilic vein, lateral antebrachial cutaneous nerve, medial antebrachial cutaneous nerve

2. flexor carpi radialis, palmaris longus, flexor digitorum superficialis, flexor pollicis longus, flexor digitorum profundus, flexor carpi ulnaris.

3. extensor carpi radialis brevis, extensor carpi radialis longus, extensor digitorum, extensor digiti minimi, extensor indicis, extensor carpi ulnaris

4. pronator teres, pronator quadratus

5. supinator, biceps brachii

6. median nerve, ulnar nerve, superficial branch of radial nerve

7. radial artery, radial vein, superficial branch of radial nerve

8. anterior interosseous nerve, anterior interosseous vessels

IV. Answer the questions briefly

1. There are five neurovascular bundles in the forearm: radial neurovascular bundle, ulnar neurovascular bundle, median neurovascular bundle and anterior interosseous neurovas-

cular bundle in anterior osteofascial compartment, posterior interosseous neurovascular bundle in posterior osteofascial compartment.

2. The radial nerve innervates the brachioradialis, the ulnar nerve innervates the flexor carpi ulnaris and the ulnar half of the flexor digitorum profundus, and the median nerve innervates the others (pronator teres, palmaris longus, flexor carpi radialis, flexor digitorum superficialis, flexor pollicis longus, pronator quadratus and radial half offlexor digitorum profundus).

V. Answer the questions in detail

1. The anterior osteofascial compartment of forearm is surrounded by deep fascia, medial intermuscular septum, lateral intermuscular septum, ulna, radius and interosseous membrane of forearm. The anterior group muscles of forearm are arranged into superficial and deep layers. Brachioradialis, pronator teres, flexor carpi radialis, palmaris longus, flexor digitorum superficialis and flexor carpi ulnaris are superficially from lateral medially; flexor pollicis longus, flexor digitorum profundus and pronator quadratus deeply. In addition, there are the radial artery, vein and nerve, the ulnar artery, vein and nerve, median nerve and accompanying vessels, the anterior interosseous artery (from common interosseous artery, a branch of ulnar artery), vein and nerve (from median nerve) in the sheath.

2. The posterior osteofascial compartment of forearm is enclosed by deep fascia, medial intermuscular septum, lateral intermuscular septum, ulna, radius and interosseous membrane of forearm. There are mainly posterior group muscles of forearm in it. These muscles are arranged into layers. Such as the extensor carpi radialis brevis, extensor carpi radialis longus, extensor digitorum, extensor digiti minimi, extensor carpi ulnaris superficially, while the supinator, abductor pollicis longus, extensor pollicis brevis, extensor pollicis longus, extensor indicis deeply. In addition, the posterior interosseous artery (from common interosseous artery, a branch of ulnar artery), vein and nerve (the terminal of deep branch of radial nerve) in the sheath.

Section 6   The Wrist and Hand

I. Single choice

   1. D   2. C   3. B   4. D   5. C   6. D   7. C   8. A   9. C   10. B

II. Double choices

   1. DE   2. AB   3. BC   4. CD   5. BD

III. Fill the blanks

   1. pisiform, hook of hamate, tubercle of scaphoid, trapezium

   2. tendon and tendinous sheath of flexor pollicis longus

   3. ulnar artery, ulnar vein, ulnar nerve

   4. tendon and tendinous sheath of abductor pollicis longus and extensor pollicis brevis,

tendon and tendinous sheath of extensor carpi radialis longus and brevis, tendon and tendinous sheath of extensor pollicis longus, tendon and tendinous sheath of extensor digitorum and indicis, tendon and tendinous sheath of extensor digiti minimi and extensor carpi ulnaris

5. midpalmar space, thenar space

IV. Answer the questions briefly

1. The carpal canal lies in front of anterior aspect of wrist and is formed by the flexor retinaculum (transverse carpal ligament) and the groove of carpal bones. The structures passing through it include the tendons of flexor digitorum superficialis and profundus in the common flexor sheath, the tendon of flexor pollicis longus in its tendinous sheath, as well as the median nerve. So carpal canal syndrome can cause injury of median nerve and result in ape palm.

2. The anatomical snuffbox is a triangular depression located on the radial side of the wrist and dorsum of the thumb. Its radial boundary is the tendons of abductor pollicis longus and extensor pollicis brevis, ulnar boundary is the tendon of extensor pollicis longus, the proximal is the styloid process of radius, the base of it is the scaphoid and the trapezium bone. The radial artery passes through and the pulsation can be touch. Fracture of scaphoid can course pain and swelling, as well as injury of radial artery.

3. The nerve supplying of skin of the hand includes the median, ulnar and radial nerves. The median nerve distributes on the palm, thenar, palmar side of radial three and a half fingers, and the dorsal side of the middle and distal digits. The ulnar nerve distributes on the hypothenar and palmar side of ulnar one and a half fingers, as well as on the ulnar half of dorsum of hand and ulnar two and a half fingers. The radial nerve distributes on the radial half of the dorsum of hand and the dorsal side of the radial two and a half fingers.

V. Answer the questions in detail

1. The layers of the palm of hand include from superficial to deep:

(1)Skin: It is thick, tight and low elastic.

(2)Superficial fascia: It is loose, but in the center of palm, it is dense and connects with the palmar aponeurosis.

(3)Superficial layer of deep fascia: It includes the palmar aponeurosis, thenar, and hypothenar fascia. The Palmar aponeurosis is a triangular shape and thickened formed by the diffuse tendinous fibers of palmaris longus. The thenar and hypothenar fascia are thin which cover the thenar and hypothenar muscles respectively.

(4)Superficial palmar arch, branches of median and ulnar nerve: The superficial palmar arch is formed by superficial palmar branch of radial artery and terminal of ulnar artery. It gives off three common palmar digital arteries and then proper palmar digital arteries companying with the branches of median and ulnar nerves same named.

(5)Deep layer of deep fascia and muscles: The deep fascia contains the palmar interosseous fascia and the fascia of adductor pollicis. There are lateral (thenar muscles), intermediate and medial (hypothenar muscles) three group muscles. The intermediate group includes the tendons of flexor digitorum superficialis and profundus, and the lumbricals.

(6)Deep palmar arch and deep branch of ulnar nerve: The deep palmar arch is formed by the terminal of radial artery and deep branch of ulnar artery, which gives off three palmar metacarpal arteries anastomosis with the common palmar arteries of the superficial palmar arch.

(7)Interosseous muscle and metacarpal bone.

2. The osteofascial compartments of the palm include three:

The lateral osteofascial compartment is formed by the lateral intermuscular septum, the thenar fascia, and 1st metacarpal bone. It contains the thenar muscles (the abductor pollicis brevis, the flexor pollicis brevis and the opponens pollicis), the tendon and tendinous sheath of flexor pollicis longus, as well as vessels and nerves of thumb.

The intermediate osteofascial compartment is enclosed by the palmar aponeurosis, the lateral intermuscular septum and medial intermuscular septum, the palmar interosseous fascia, and the fascia of adductor pollicis. It contains the tendons of flexor digit (superficialis and profundus) and its common sheath, the lumbricals, superficial palmar arch, and its branches, as well as branches of median and ulnar nerves.

The medial osteofascial compartment is enclosed by the hypothenar fascia, the medial intermuscular septum, and the 5th metacarpal bone. It includes the hypothenar muscles (the abductor digiti minimi, the flexor digiti minimi brevis and opponens digiti minimi), the vessels and nerves of little finger.

Chapter 4   The Lower Limb

Section 1 Introduction

Ⅰ. Single choice

1. C 2. B 3. D

Ⅱ. Double choices

1. AC 2. BE 3. BC

Ⅲ. Fill the blanks

1. the gluteal region, the thigh, the leg, the foot

2. dorsal artery

3. anterior tibial artery

4. the sciatic nerve

IV. Answer the questions briefly

1. The lower limb is directly anchored to the trunk. It is bounded anteriorly by the inguinal groove that connected with abdomen, and posteriorly by iliac crest that connected with the waist and sacrum. Between the medial sides of the upper extremities of the two lower limbs is the perineum.

2. The lower limb can be divided into following parts: the gluteal region, the thigh, the leg and the foot. Besides the gluteal region, the other parts are divided into different regions.

3. The iliac crest ends anteriorly as the anterior superior iliac spine and posteriorly as the posterior superior iliac spine. The tubercle of iliac crest, the greater trochanter, the symphysis pubis, the pubic crest, the pubic tubercle, and the inguinal ligament.

4. The medial malleolus, the lateral malleolus, the tendo calcaneus, the calcaneal tuberosity, the tuberosity of the navicular bone and the fifth metatarsal bone.

5. They leave the pelvis near the midpoint of the line joining the posterior superior iliac spine and the ischial tuberosity.

Section 2   The Gluteal Region

I. Single choice

1. C   2. B   3. D   4. D   5. A   6. C   7. A   8. B   9. C   10. A

II. Double choices

1. AC   2. BE   3. BD   4. AD   5. CE   6. AB   7. DE

III. Fill the blanks

1. The posterior branch of lateral femoral cutaneous nerve

2. lower part of the buttock

3. Gluteal maximus

4. Piriformis, greater sciatic foramen

5. internal iliac artery

IV. Answer the questions briefly

1. The superficial blood vessels of the gluteal region include the cutaneous artery and musculocutaneous artery. They are the branches of the 4th lumbar artery, the inferior gluteal artery, and the lateral sacral artery. The superficial veins accompany the corresponding superficial arteries. The lymph vessels of the gluteal region drain into the lateral group of the superficial inguinal lymph nodes.

2. The cutaneous nerves of the gluteal region include the subcostal nerve, the lateral cutaneous branch of iliohypogastric nerve, the posterior branch of lateral femoral cutaneous nerve, the inferior cluneal nerves, the superior cluneal nerves and the medial cluneal nerves.

V. Answer the questions in detail

1. The sciatic nerve arises from the sacral plexus and passes through infrapiriform foramen into the gluteal region, deep to gluteus maximus, passing midway between thegreater

trochanter of femur and ischial tuberosity to back of thigh, the nerve lies deep to the long head of biceps on the posterior surface of adductor magnus. The sciatic nerve usually ends half-way down the back of the thigh by dividing into the common peroneal and tibial nerves. The sciatic nerve to supply the semitendinosus, semimembranosus and biceps femoris. It has articular branches to supply the hip and knee joints. Occasionally, the sciatic nerve divides into its two terminal parts at a higher level, in the upper part of the thigh, the gluteal region or even inside the pelvis.

2. The blood vessels and nerves which pass through the suprapiriform foramen are arranged from the lateral to the medial side as follows: the superior gluteal nerve, the superior gluteal artery, and the vein. The superior gluteal artery is a branch of internal iliac artery. As it emerges from the suprapiriform foramen, it divided immediately into superficial and deep branches. The superficial branch supplies the gluteus maximus; its deep branch supplies the gluteus medius and minimus and the tensor fasciae latae. It anastomoses with the inferior gluteal and lateral femoral circumflex arteries. The superior gluteal vein drains into the internal iliac vein. The superior gluteal nerve is a branch of sacral plexus; it runs between the gluteus medius and minimus with the deep branch of superior gluteal artery and supplies these two muscles and the tensor fasciae latae.

3. The blood vessels and nerves which pass through the infrapiriform foramen are arranged from the lateral to the medial side as follows: the sciatic nerve, the posterior femoral cutaneous nerve, the inferior gluteal nerve, the inferior gluteal artery and vein, the internal pudendal artery and vein, and the pudendal nerve. The inferior gluteal artery is another branch of the internal iliac artery; it chiefly supplies the gluteus maxims and anastomoses with the superior gluteal artery, the first perforating branch of deep femoral artery and the medial and lateral femoral circumflex arteries. It also gives off branches to the hip joint. The inferior gluteal nerve is a branch of the sacral plexus. As it emerges from the infrapiriform foramina, the nerve immediately breaks up into several branches to supply the overlying gluteus maximus. The posterior femoral cutaneous nerve, a branch of sacral plexus, emerges from the infrapiriform foramen on the posterior surface of the sciatic nerve, then it descends along the median line of the back of the thigh. Its branches supply the skin of inferior part of the buttock, the back of the thigh, popliteal region and the upper part of the leg. Its perineal branch passes medially to the scrotum or greater lip of pudendum.

Section 3　The Thigh

Ⅰ. **Single choice**

1. A　2. B　3. D　4. D　5. B　6. D　7. B　8. C　9. C　10. D　11. A　12. C　13. B 14. B　15. A　16. D　17. C　18. C　19. B　20. B

Ⅱ. **Double choices**

1. AB　2. BC　3. AD　4. BE　5. BD　6. CE　7. CD　8. BD　9. DE　10. AD

Ⅲ. Fill the blanks

1. fatty layer, membranous layer
2. superficial epigastric, superficial iliac circumflex, external pudendal
3. saphenous nerve
4. iliotibial tract
5. sartorius, quadriceps femoris
6. Femoral artery, Femoral vein
7. adductor longus, pectineus, iliopsoas
8. Femoral canal
9. femoral ring
10. lateral circumflex artery, medial circumflex artery, perforating arteries
11. lumbar plexus
12. obturator canal
13. biceps femoris, semitendinosus, semimembranosus
14. tibial nerve, common peroneal nerve
15. Great saphenous vein

Ⅳ. Answer the questions briefly

1. The lacuna musculorum is bounded by lateral portion of inguinal ligament anteriorly, ilium posterolaterally, iliopectineal arch medially. It contains the iliopsoas, femoral nerve and the lateral femoral cutaneous nerve.

2. The posterior osteofascial compartment of the thigh contains the biceps femoris, semitendinosus, semimembranosus, branches of the deep femoral artery and the sciatic nerve.

3. The lacuna vasorum is bounded by medial portion of inguinal ligament anteriorly, pectineal ligament posteromedially, lacunar ligament medially and iliopectineal arch posterolaterally. It contains the femoral sheath, genital branch of genitofemoral nerve and lymphatic vessels.

4. The femoral sheath derived from transverse fascia anteriorly and iliac fascia posteriorly. The femoral artery occupies the lateral compartment of the sheath. The femoral vein lies the middle compartment. The medial compartment is small, called the femoral canal.

5. The adduct canal is bounded by vastus medialis laterally, adductors longus and magnus posteriorly, and adductor lamina and sartorius anteriorly. It contains thesaphenous nerve, femoral artery, femoral vein, lymphatic vessels and loose connective tissue.

Ⅴ. Answer the questions in detail

1. The femoral triangle is bounded by inguinal ligament above, medial border of sartorius laterally, and medial border of adductor longus medially. Anterior wall is formed fascia lata. Posterior wall is formed by iliopsoas, pectineus, adductor longus and their fascia. It contains the femoral nerve, femoral artery, femoral vein and femoral canal compartmentalized

within the femoral sheath. The femoral sheath surrounds the femoral vessels and lymphatic about 2. 5 cm below the inguinal ligament. Its lower end disappears at the lower margin of the saphenous opening where the sheath fuses with the adventitia of the vessels. The femoral artery occupies the lateral compartment of the sheath. The femoral vein lies the middle compartment. The femoral canal is the medial compartment of the femoral sheath, about 1. 5 cm long and contains a little loose fatty tissue, a small lymph node and some lymph vessels.

The femoral artery is the main artery of the lower limb and is directly continuous with the external iliac artery of the abdomen behind the inguinal ligament at the mid-inguinal point. It becomes the popliteal artery by passing through the adductor tendinous opening. It gives off lateral circumflex artery, medial circumflex artery, and three perforating arteries. The femoral vein is the direct continuation of the popliteal vein. The deep inguinal lymph nodes lie medial to the femoral vein. The femoral nerve arises from the lumbar plexus in the abdomen and enters the thigh posterior to the inguinal ligament and lateral to the femoral artery. It ends by dividing into a number of branches 2 cm below the inguinal ligament.

2. The great saphenous vein is the largest and thickest walled superficial vein of the lower limb. It begins on the medial side of the dorsum of the foot and runs upwards anteriorly to the medial malleolus and then on the medial surface of the leg, accompanying with the saphenous nerve. It then ascends on the posteromedial surface of the knee and inclines anteriorly through the thigh to enter the femoral vein through the saphenous hiatus. On its course, the great saphenous vein receives superficial veins of the leg and other five tributaries: the superficial epigastric vein, the superficial iliaccircumflex vein, the external pudendal vein, the superficial medial femoral vein and the superficial lateral femoral vein. All the tributaries vary greatly in number, site and type draining into the great saphenous vein. The vein and its some tributaries have several communications through the deep fascia with the deep veins, particularly in region of the ankle and knee. Most of these communications are guarded by valves which prevent reflux of blood from the deep veins.

Section 4　The Knee

Ⅰ. Single choice
　　1. A　2. A　3. D　4. B　5. D　6. D　7. B　8. D　9. C　10. C

Ⅱ. Double choices
　　1. BC　2. BE　3. BC　4. AB

Ⅲ. Fill the blanks
　　1. medial meniscus, lateral meniscus
　　2. anterior cruciate ligament, posterior cruciate ligament
　　3. popliteal artery
　　4. popliteal fascia

IV. Answer the questions briefly

1. The popliteal vein is formed by the junction of the venae concomitants of the anterior and posterior tibial arteries at the lower border of the popliteus on the medial side of the popliteal artery. As it ascends through the fossa, it crosses behind the popliteal artery, so that it comes to lie on its lateral side. It passes through the adductor tendinous opening to become the femoral vein.

2. The common peroneal nerve gives off articular branches to the knee and proximal tibiofibular joints. It also gives off the lateral sural cutaneous nerve to the skin of the calf and the lateral side of the back of the leg and a communicating branch which joints the sural nerve.

3. The tibial nerve gives off three genicular branches. It also gives off cutaneous and muscular branches in the distal part of the fossa. The cutaneous branch is called the medial sural cutaneous nerve which supplies the skin of the calf and the back of the leg and joint with the communicating branch of common peroneal nerve to form the sural nerve which supplies the lateral aspect of the ankle and the foot. The muscular branches supply the gastrocnemius, plantaris, soleus and popliteus.

4. The popliteal artery is deeply placed and enters the popliteal fossa through the adductor tendinous opening, as a continuation of the femoral artery. It ends at the level of the lower border of the popliteus by dividing into anterior and posterior tibial arteries. The branches of popliteal artery are cutaneous, muscular and articular to supply the skin on the posterior aspect of the leg, the knee joint and the muscles surrounding the popliteal fossa.

V. Answer the questions in detail

The popliteal fossa is a diamond-shaped intermuscular space situated at the back of the knee. The fossa is most prominent when the knee joint is flexed. It contains the popliteal vessels, the small saphenous vein, the common peroneal and tibial nerves, the posterior cutaneous nerve of the thigh, the genicular branch of the obturator nerve, connective tissue, and lymph nodes. The upper lateral boundary is formed by the bicepsfemoris and the upper medial boundary by the semitendinosus and semimembranosus. The lower lateral boundary is formed by the lateral head of the gastrocnemius and the lower media boundary by the medial head of the gastrocnemius. The floor of the fossa is formed from above downwards by the popliteal surface of femur, the posterior capsule of the knee joint and the popliteus with its fascia. The roof of the popliteal fossa is formed by the popliteal fascia. The tibial nerve runs vertically through the popliteal fossa, posterior to the popliteal vessels. The common peroneal nerve runs along the medial border of the biceps femoris to the back of the head of the fibula. It then curves forwards between the neck of the fibula and the upper fibers of the peroneus longus. Here the nerve divides into superficial and deep peroneal nerves. The popliteal vein formed by the junction of the anterior and posterior tibial veins near the lower border of the popliteus. The deep popliteal lymph nodes just under the deep fascia, close to the popliteal fossa vessels. The popliteal artery enters the popliteal fossa through the opening in the adductor magnus, as a continuous of the femoral artery. It ends at the lower border of the popliteus where it divides into anterior tibial artery and posterior tibial artery.

Section 5   The Leg

I . Single choice

1. B   2. D   3. C   4. B   5. C   6. B   7. B   8. D   9. A   10. D   11. A   12. C   13. B
14. B   15. A   16. B   17. A   18. D   19. A   20. A

II . Double choices

1. AC   2. AB   3. CD   4. CD   5. AB

III . Fill the blanks

1. dorsal venous arch, saphenous nerve

2. peroneus longus, peroneus brevis, superficial peroneal nerve

3. tibialis anterior, extensor hallucis longus, extensor digitorum longus, deep peroneal nerve

4. small saphenous vein, sural nerve

5. gastrocnemius, soleus

6. saphenous nerve, femoral nerve

7. gastrocnemius, plantaris, soleus, popliteus, tibialis posterior, flexor hallucis longus, flexor digitorum longus

8. medial sural cutaneous nerve, lateral sural cutaneous nerve, sural nerve

IV . Answer the questions briefly

1. In the anterior osteofascial compartment of leg, there are three muscles, three blood vessels, and one nerve. They are tibialis anterior, extensor hallucis longus, extensor digitorum longus, anterior tibial artery, two anterior tibial veins and deep peroneal nerve.

2. In the lateral osteofascial compartment of leg, there are two muscles and one nerve. They are peroneus longus, peroneus brevis and superficial peroneal nerve.

3. In the medial side of leg, there are great saphenous vein and saphenous nerve; in the lateral side of leg, there is superficial peroneal nerve; in the back of leg, there are small saphenous vein, medial sural cutaneous nerve, lateral sural cutaneous nerve and sural nerve.

V . Answer the questions in detail

In the posterior osteofascial compartment of leg, there are muscles, blood vessels and nerves. The muscles are divides into two layers (superficial and deep layers) by the deep transverse fascia. The superficial layer contains gastrocnemius, plantaris and soleus. The deep layer contains popliteus, tibialis posterior, flexor hallucis longus and flexor digitorum longus. Between these two layers of muscles, there are the posterior tibial artery, tibial nerve and two posterior tibial veins.

Section 6   The Ankle and Foot

I . Single choice

1. B   2. C   3. D   4. A   5. B   6. D   7. C   8. C

II . Double choices

1. AC   2. BE   3. DE   4. DE

III. Fill the blanks

1. medial malleolus, calcaneus, flexor retinaculum

2. tendon and synovial sheath of tibialis posterior, tendon and synovial sheath of flexor digitorum longus, posterior tibial vessels, and tibial nerve, tendon and synovial sheath of flexor hallucis longus

3. medial plantar artery, lateral plantar artery

4. medial plantar nerve, lateral plantar nerve

5. tibialis anterior, extensor hallucis longus, extensor digitorum longus

IV. Answer the questions briefly

1. There are five cutaneous nerves on the dorsum of foot. The saphenous nerve supplies the skin along the medial side of the foot. The cutaneous branch of deep peroneal nerve supplies the skin of the adjacent sides of the big and second toes. The lateral dorsal cutaneous nerve (terminal branch of sural nerve) supplies the skin along the lateral side of the foot. Other regions are innervated by the medial and intermediate dorsal cutaneous nerves.

2. The malleolar canal is formed by medial malleolus, calcaneus and flexor retinaculum. From anterior posteriorly, the structures passing through the malleolar canal are the tendon and synovial sheath of tibialis posterior, tendon and synovial sheath of flexor digitorum longus, posterior tibial vessels and tibial nerve, tendon and synovial sheath of flexor hallucis longus.

Chapter 5   The Thorax

Section 1   Introduction

I . Single choice

B

II . Double choices

CE

Ⅲ. Fill the blanks

7th to 10th

Section 2　The Thoracic Wall

Ⅰ. Single choice

1. D　2. B　3. B　4. B　5. A　6. D　7. B　8. B　9. C　10. A

Ⅱ. Double choices

1. AB　2. AD　3. CE　4. CD　5. BC

Ⅲ. Fill the blanks

1. cephalic vein, thoracoacromial artery, thoracoacromial vein, lateral pectoral nerve

2. posterior intercostal vein, posterior intercostal artery, intercostal nerve

Ⅳ. Answer the questions briefly

1. The clavipectoral fascia is a strong fibrous sheet, extending between the pectoralis minor and subciavians. It is pierced by cephalic vein, thoracoacromial artery and vein and lateral pectoral nerve.

2. The muscles: the intercostales externi, the intercostales interni and intercostales intimi.

The posteriorintercostal artery, posterior intercostal vein and intercostal nerve lay between the intercostales interni and intercostales intimi. In the costal groove of the rib, the arrangement from up downwards is the vein, artery and nerve.

3. The female breast lies superficial the pectoral fascia, overlies the 2nd to 6th or 7th ribs between the parasternal line and middle axillary line.

The female breast is composed of skin, fatty tissue, fibrous tissue and mammary gland.

Ⅴ. Answer the questions in detail

1. Most of the lymphatic vessels of the female breast drain into the axillary lymph nodes. Some of them drain into the parasternal lymph nodes and pectoral lymph nodes.

(1) superficial lymphatic vessels: no valves and forms the plexus, drain into the deep lymphatic vessels or pectoral lymph nodes (anterior group of the axillary lymph nodes).

(2) deep lymphatic vessels: have valves and diameter is more larger, drain into:

1) lateral and upper parts—pectoral lymph nodes—apical lymph nodes.

2) medial part—the parasternal lymph nodes—anterior mediastinal lymph nodes or supraclavicular lymph nodes, or forms the anastomoses with the vessels of the opposite side.

3) inferomedial part—anastomose with the vessels of the anterior abdominal wall and with the subdiaphragmatic and hepatic lymph vessels.

4) Deep part—lymph nodes between the pectoralis major and minor and deep to the pectoralis minor—the apical lymph nodes.

2. The skin of the anterior thoracic wall above the second rib is supplied by the supraclavicular nerves. The area below this level is supplied by the anterior cutaneous branches of the

intercostal nerves. The distribution of the anterior branches of the 12 pairs of thoracic nerves is segmental. On the anterior surface of the trunk, they present about the levels as follows:

T_2— the sternal angle, T_4— the nipple, T_6— the xiphoid process,

T_8— the lowest of the costal arch, T_{10}— the umbilicus,

T_{12}— the anterior superior iliac spine.

Section 3   The Pleura, Pleural Cavity and Lungs

Ⅰ. Single choice

1. C   2. D   3. B   4. D   5. C   6. A   7. C   8. B   9. D   10. A

Ⅱ. Double choices

1. AE   2. BC   3. AD   4. BC   5. CE

Ⅲ. Fill the blanks

1. pulmonary vein, pulmonary artery, bronchus

2. (superior lobar) bronchus, pulmonary artery, the (middle and inferior lobar) bronchi, pulmonary vein

3. parietal, visceral pleura

4. costodiaphragmatic recess

5. triangle of pericardium

Ⅳ. Answer the questions briefly

1. The pleura is a thin layer of serous membrane covering the surface of the lungs and lining to the inner surface of the thoracic cage. It has two parts: the parietal and visceral pleura.

The parietal pleura is the portion lining to the inner surface of the thoracic cage. It can be divided into 4 parts according to their covering location: the cupula of pleura, costal pleura, diaphragmatic pleura and mediastinal pleura.

2. The pleural cavity is a potential space between the parietal pleura and visceral pleura. It contains a capillary layer of serous lubricating fluid.

The pleural recesses, formed by two different parts of the parietal pleura, can't be occupied by the expanded lung, and they are costodiaphragmatic recess and the costomediastinal recess, as well as diaphragmatic recess (only on the left side).

3. The chief structures composing the root of each lung are arranged in a similar manner from anterior to posterior on both sides; they are the pulmonary vein, the pulmonary artery and the bronchus, with the bronchial vessels on its posterior aspect behind. However, their arrangement differs from above downwards. On the right, their arrangement is superior lobar bronchus, pulmonary artery, middle and inferior lobar bronchus and pulmonary vein; on the left, they are the pulmonary artery, the bronchus and the pulmonary vein.

4. The lower border of the pleura commences from the back of the 6th sternocostal joint

of the right side and from the midpoint of the 6th costal cartilage on the left. Then it passes obliquely across the 8th rib in the midclavicular line, the 10th rib in the midaxillary line and the 12th rib in the scapular line.

5. The superior vena cava and the right atrium lie in front of the root of the right lung, and the azygos vein arch above it. The root of the left lung is ventral to the thoracic aorta and inferior to the aortic arch. The phrenic nerves, the pericardiacophrenic vessels and the anterior pulmonary plexuses of nerves lie ventral to both roots of the lungs. The vagus nerve and the posterior pulmonary plexuses lie dorsal to the roots on both sides.

V. Answer the questions in detail

1. The sternal reflection is where the costal pleura is continuous with the mediastinal pleura behind the sternum. The right and left sternal reflections are indicated by lines that pass inferiomedially from the sternoclavicular joints to the median line at the level of the sternal angle, here the two pleura sac come in contact and may slightly overlap each other. On the right side, the reflection continues downwards in the midline to the back of the 6th sternocostal joint. On the left side, the reflection passed downwards in the midline to the level of the 4th costal cartilage, then it deviates to the left and descends obliquely, posterior to the 4th to 5th intercostal spaces, 2.5 cm apart from the left margin of sternum. At the midpoint of the 6th costal cartilage, it continues with its costal reflection. Above the sternal angle and below the level of the 4th costal cartilage, the distance between two sternal reflections is larger. The superior intermediate region is called the triangle of thymus, and the inferior is the triangle of pericardium.

The costal reflection is where the costal pleura is continuous with the diaphragmatic pleura. It commences from the back of the 6th sternocostal joint of the right side and from the midpoint of the 6th costal cartilage on the left. Then it passes obliquely across the 8th rib in the midclavicular line, the 10th rib in the midaxillary line and the 12th rib in the scapular line.

2. The lungs occupy most space in the thoracic cavity, and they are separated by the mediastinum, mainly the heart and large blood vessels.

Each lung has the shape of a half cone andpresents an apex, a base, two surfaces and three borders. The apex extends into the root of the neck 3 – 5 cm above the anterior part of the first rib and 2 cm above the medial one-third of the clavicle. The base of the lung is semilunar in shape. It is fitted to the dome of the diaphragm and so deeply concave, especially on the right side where the dome is higher than the left. The anterior border is thin and overlaps the pericardium. There is a cardiac notch at the anterior border of the left lung. The posterior border is thick and rounded. The inferior border is sharp and semilunar in shape. The costal surface is large, smooth and convex. The mediastinal surface is towards the mediastinum and the hilum of the lung lies near the center of this surface.

The left lung is divided into two lobes by a deep oblique fissure. The right lung is divided into the superior, middle and inferior lobes by the oblique fissure and the horizontal fissure.

There are some structures passing through the hilum of the lung. The chief structures are arranged in a similar manner from anterior to the posterior on both sides: the pulmonary vein, the pulmonary artery and the bronchus. Their arrangement differs from above downwards on the two sides: on the right, they are the superior lobar bronchus, the pulmonary artery, middle and inferior lobar bronchi and the pulmonary vein; on the left, they are the pulmonary artery, the bronchus and the pulmonary vein.

Section 4 The Diaphragm

Ⅰ. Single choice

1. D   2. B

Ⅱ. Double choices

1. BE   2. AB

Ⅲ. Fill the blanks

1. sternal, costal, lumbar

2. 12th, azygos vein, thoracic duct

Ⅳ. Answer the questions briefly

There are three openings of the diaphragm as below.

(1) The aortic hiatus is at the level of 12th thoracic vertebra, slightly to the left of the median plane. The aorta, azygos vein and thoracic duct transmit the hiatus.

(2) The esophageal hiatus is located in the right crus of the diaphragm, 2 – 3 cm to the left of the median plane, at the level of the 10th thoracic vertebra. The esophagus and two vagal trunks pass through the hiatus.

(3) The vena caval foramen is located in the central tendon of the diaphragm, at the level of 8th thoracic vertebra, 2 – 3 cm to the right of the median plane. The inferior vena cava, the terminal branches of right phrenic nerve pass through it.

Section 5 The Mediastinum

Ⅰ. Single choice

1. D   2. B   3. A   4. C   5. A   6. B   7. D   8. C   9. C   10. D   11. A   12. D   13. B   14. C   15. A

Ⅱ. Double choices

1. AB   2. CE   3. BD   4. AB   5. BC   6. AD   7. DE   8. CE

Ⅲ. Fill the blanks

1. internal jugular vein, the subclavian vein

2. the brachiocephalic trunk, the left common carotid artery, the left subclavian artery

3. great splanchnic nerve

4. cisterna chyli

5. root of the right lung, superior vena cava

IV. Answer the questions briefly

1. There are 3 layers in the superior mediastinum.

Superficial layer: thymus and three veins (left brachiocephalic v., right brachiocephalic v. and superior vena cava);

Middle layer: aortic arch and its three branches, phrenic n. and vagus n.;

Deep layer: trachea, esophagus, thoracic duct and left recurrent laryngeal n.

2. The triangle of the ductus arteriosus is formed by the left pulmonary artery inferiorly, the left phrenic nerve anteriorly and the left vagus nerve posteriorly.

The arterial ligamentthe left recurrent laryngeal nerve and the superficial cardiac plexuses lie in the triangle of the ductus arteriosus.

3. Anteriorly, the esophagus is in relation with the trachea, left recurrent laryngeal nerve, left principal bronchus, pericardium, and diaphragm. Posterior to the esophagus, there are the right posterior intercostal arteries, azygos, hemiazygos veins, the inferior part of the thoracic duct and the loose connective tissue. On the left side, the esophagus is related to the left common carotid artery, left subclavian artery, aortic arch, thoracic aorta, the superior part of the thoracic duct and the left mediastinal pleura, etc. On the right side, there are azygos vein and its arch, and right mediastinal pleura.

4. The retroesophageal space is located between the esophagus and the intrathoracic fascia within the superior mediastinum. There are the thoracic duct, azygos and hemiazygos veins in the space. It connects with the retropharyngeal space superiorly, and the retroperitoneal space through the hiatus of the diaphragm inferiorly.

V. Answer the questions in detail

1. There is the root of the left lung is the center on the left surface of the mediastinum. The aortic arch is above, the left phrenic nerve and pericardiacophrenic vessels in front, and the thoracic aorta behind. The esophagus lies behind the left subclavian artery, where the esophagus slightly inclines to the left side. The thoracic duct clings to the left aspect of the esophagus. Behind the esophagus and the thoracic aorta, there is the thoracic part of the sympathetic trunk, thoracic sympathetic ganglia and greater splanchnic, descending on the left side of the thoracic vertebrae and lateral to the accessory hemiazygos and hemiazygos veins. The left vagus nerve lies to the left of the aortic arch and then runs downwards between the root of the lung and the thoracic aorta. Under the root of the lung, between the pericardium and thoracic aorta, the esophagus appears to the right of the left vagus nerve.

2. **Location:** The esophagus commences in the neck at the median plane and deviates slightly to the left as it approaches the thoracic inlet. The thoracic part of the esophagus descends in front of the vertebral column in the superior and posterior mediastinum, passes

through the esophageal hiatus of the diaphragm, and then become the abdominal part of the esophagus. At the inlet of the thorax, the esophagus lies between the trachea and thoracic vertebrae and deviates slightly to the left. At the level of the tracheal bifurcation, it lies in median plane posterior to the bifurcation and anterior and left to the azygos vein. Under the azygos arch, the esophagus slightly deviates to the left. At the level of the 10th thoracic vertebra, the esophagus passes through the esophagus hiatus of the diaphragm and become to the abdominal part of the esophagus.

Relations: Anteriorly, the esophagus is in relation with the trachea, left recurrent laryngeal nerve, left principal bronchus, pericardium, and diaphragm. Posterior to the esophagus, there are the right posterior intercostal arteries, azygos, hemiazygos veins, the inferior part of the thoracic duct and the loose connective tissue. On the left side, the esophagus is related to the left common carotid artery, left subclavian artery, aortic arch, thoracic aorta, the superior part of the thoracic duct and the left mediastinal pleura, etc. On the right side, there are azygos vein and its arch, and right mediastinal pleura.

Blood supply: The superior segment of the thoracic part of the esophagus is supplied by the first, second posterior intercostal arteries, the esophageal branch of the inferior thyroid artery, the costocervical trunk and bronchial artery; the inferior segment is supplied by the esophageal branch of the thoracic aorta and the 4th – 7th posterior intercostal arteries. The veins accompany the arteries. The most veins of the esophagus enter into the posterior intercostal veins and then drain into the hemiazygos vein, azygous vein. The veins of the inferior part of esophagus enter into the left gastric vein and then drain into the hepatic portal vein.

Lymphatic drainage: The lymph of the superior part of the esophagus drains into the anterior mediastinal and the tracheobronchial lymph nodes; the middle part drains to the periesophageal pulmonary and posterior mediastinal lymph nodes; the inferior part drains into the left gastric and celiac lymph nodes. In addition, some lymph of the esophagus directly drains into the thoracic duct.

Chapter 6   The Abdomen

Section 1   Introduction

Ⅰ. **Single choice**

    1. D   2. C   3. B

Ⅱ. **Double choices**

    1. AD   2. AC   3. CE

III. Fill the blanks

1. abdominal wall, abdominal cavity, abdominal organs

2. diaphragm, the superior orifice of the pelvic cavity

3. linea semilunar

4. 3rd, 4th

5. inferior mesenteric

Section 2　The Anterolateral Abdominal Wall

I. Single choice

1. A　2. C　3. D　4. D　5. C　6. D　7. A　8. A　9. C　10. D　11. C　12. B　13. D
14. D　15. B　16. C　17. B　18. A　19. B　20. D　21. D　22. D　23. B　24. A　25. A

II. Double choices

1. BE　2. BD　3. CE　4. CD　5. BD

III. Fill the blanks

1. camper fascia (fatty layer), scapa fascia (membranous layer)

2. the sixth intercostal nerve, the tenth intercostal nerve

3. superficial iliac circumflex artery, superficial epigastric artery, femoral artery

4. thoracoepigastric vein, axillary vein

5. superficial iliac circumflex vein, superficial epigastric vein

6. axillary lymph nodes, superficial inguinal lymph nodes

7. rectus abdominis, obliquus externus abdominis, obliquus internus abdominis, transversus abdominis

8. spermatic cord, round ligament of uterus

9. superior epigastric artery, inferior epigastric artery

10. lateral margin of rectus abdominis, inguinal ligament, inferior epigastric vessels

IV. Answer the questions briefly

1. The median incision is along the anterior median line. The paramedian incision is placed 2. 5 – 4. 0 cm lateral and parallel to the median line. The rectus incisionis the same as the paramedian incision but with an additional incision of the rectus abdominis. The pararectal incision is made along the lateral side of the rectus abdominis. The subcostal incision is used to the right side in biliary surgery and on the left in exposure of the spleen. The McBurney's incision is an oblique incision centered at the McBurney's point. In addition, there are the transverse incision, oblique incision and so on.

2. The layers are as follows from superficial to deep: skin, superficial fascia, obliquus externus abdominis, obliquus internus abdominis, transversus abdominis, transverse fascia, extraperitoneal fascia and parietal peritoneum.

3. It can form inguinal ligament, lateral and medial crura, lacunar ligament, reflected

ligament, superficial ring of the inguinal canal, anterior wall of inguinal canal, anterior sheath of rectus abdominis, pectineal ligament, external spermatic fascia, etc.

4. There are several arteries in the deep structures of the anterolateral abdominal wall. The lower 5 pairs of posterior intercostal artery and subcostal artery arise from the abdominal aorta and supply blood to muscles in the abdominal wall. The superior epigastric artery arises from the internal thoracic artery and goes downwards deep to the rectus abdominis. The inferior epigastric artery and deep iliac circumflex artery originate from the external iliac artery and supply the lower part of the abdominal wall.

V. Answer the questions in detail

1. The inguinal canal is an oblique passage about 4 cm in length passing downwards and medially from the deep to the superficial inguinal rings. The inguinal canal lies parallel to and immediately above the inguinal ligament. It has four walls and two openings.

The anterior wall is formed by the aponeurosis of obliquus externus abdominis, andlaterally is reinforced by the muscular fibers of obliquus internus abdominis. Its posterior wall is formed by the transverse fascia and the inguinal flax. The superior wall is formed by the arched fibers of the obliquus internus abdominis and the transversus abdominis. Its inferior wall is formed by the inguinal ligament.

The deep inguinal ring lies at a fingerbreadth above the midpoint of the inguinal ligament and formed by the transverse fascia. The superficial inguinal ring lies adjacent to the pubic tubercle and formed by the aponeurosis of obliquus externus abdominis.

The inguinal canal contains the spermatic cord in male or the round ligament in female and the ilioinguinal nerve in both.

2. The rectus sheath is formed by three layers of aponeurosis of the lateral group muscles in the abdominal wall, and it encloses the rectus abdominis. Above the level 4 cm below the umbilicus, the anterior wall of sheath is formed by the aponeurosis of the obliquus externus abdominis and the anterior layer of the obliquus internus abdominis aponeurosis. The posterior wall of the sheath is formed by the posterior layer of the obliquus internus abdominis aponeurosis and the aponeurosis of the transversus abdominis. Its inferior margin is named the arcuate line.

Below the level 4 cm below the umbilicus, the anterior wall of sheath is formed by the three layers of aponeurosis, and the posterior wall of sheath is lack.

Section 3　The Peritoneum and Peritoneal Cavity

I. Single choice

1. B　2. B　3. C　4. B　5. D　6. A　7. B　8. D　9. B　10. D

II. Double choices

1. AC　2. BC　3. AD　4. BE　5. CE

Ⅲ. Fill the blanks

1. omentum, mesentery, ligament
2. hepatogastric ligament, hepatoduodunal ligament
3. hepatorenal recess
4. omental foramen
5. intra-peritoneal organs, meso-peritoneal organs, extra-peritoneal organs

Ⅳ. Answer the questions briefly

1. The omental bursa lies behind the stomach and the lesser omentum. Its superior wall is the inferior surface of the caudate lobe of the liver and a part of the peritoneum covering the diaphragm. It inferior wall is the transverse colon and its mesocolon. The anterior wall is formed by the lesser omentum, the posterior wall of stomach and gastrocolic ligament. The posterior wall is formed by the peritoneum covering the pancreas, left kidney and left suprarenal gland. On the left, it is bounded by the spleen, the gastrosplenic and splenorenal ligament. On the right, it communicates with greater sac by the omental foramen.

2. The ligaments formed by peritoneum of liver include the left and right triangular ligaments, right and left coronary ligaments, the falciform ligament, hepatogastric ligament and hepatoduodenal ligament. In addition, the ligament formed by peritoneum in supracolic compartment has gastrosplenic ligament, gastrocolic ligament, splenorenal ligament, phrenicosplenic ligament and so on.

3. The organs in abdominal cavityare divided into three groups according to the covering of the peritoneum. The intra-peritoneal organs are almost completely covered by peritoneum and more mobile than others are, such as stomach, spleen, jejunum, ileum, cecum, etc. The meso-peritoneal organs are covered by peritoneum on three aspects, such as gallbladder, liver, uterus, ascending colon, etc. The extro-peritoneal organs are covered by peritoneum only on one aspect, such as kidney, pancreas, suprarenal gland and son on.

Ⅴ. Answer the questions in detail

The peritoneal cavity can be divided into supracolic and infracolic compartments by the transverse colon and its mesocolon. Supracolic compartment lies between the diaphragm and the transverse mesocolon, and infracolic compartment lies below the transverse mesocolon.

In supracolic compartment (also named subphrenic space), the space include the left anterior suprahepatic space, left posterior suprahepatic space, right suprahepatic space, right infrahepatic space (also named hepatorenal recess), left anterior infrahepatic space and left posterior infrahepatic space (omental bursa).

In infracolic compartment, there are four spaces: the right and left paracolic sulci, the right and left mesenteric sinuses.

Section 4 The Supracolic Compartment

I. Single choice

1. D 2. C 3. A 4. C 5. D 6. A 7. C 8. D 9. B 10. C 11. C 12. D 13. C
14. D 15. A 16. C 17. B 18. D 19. A 20. B

II. Double choices

1. BD 2. AE 3. BE 4. AB 5. AB 6. AC 7. CE 8. CD 9. BC 10. BE

III. Fill the blanks

1. right gastroepiploic artery, left gastroepiploic artery

2. sympathetic, parasympathetic

3. left lobe of liver, diaphragm, anterior abdominal wall

4. superior duodenal flexure; inferior duodenal flexure; duodenojejunal flexure (suspensory ligament of duodenum)

5. superficial iliac circumflex vein, superficial epigastric vein

6. superior mesenteric vessels, the root of mesentery

7. fissure for ligamentum teres hepatis, fissure for ligamentum venosum; fossa for gallbladder, sulcus for inferior vena cava

8. cystic duct, common hepatic duct, inferior surface of the liver

9. fundus, body, neck, cystic duct

10. major duodenal papilla

11. head

12. minor duodenal papilla

13. splenic notch

14. celiac trunk, body of pancreas

15. gastrosplenic ligament, phrenicosplenic ligament, splenorenal ligament

IV. Answer the questions briefly

1. The porta hepatis (or the first porta hepatis) is the cross-bar of "H" shaped grooves. At the porta hepatis, there are the branches of the hepatic portal vein, the right and left branches of the proper hepatic artery, the right and left hepatic ducts, the hepatic nerve plexus and lymphatic vessels entering or leaving the liver. In the superior margin of the sulcus for vena cava lies the second porta hepatis where the right, left and intermediate hepatic veins leave the liver and enter into the inferior vena cava. In the inferior part of the sulcus for the vena cava, there is the third porta hepatis.

2. The spleen is located in the left hypochondriac region of abdomen. It lies obliquely with its long axis and parallels with the 9th, 10th and 11th ribs.

The diaphragmatic surface faces the diaphragm; the visceral surface is adjacent to the stomach, left kidney, left colic flexure and tail of pancreas.

3. Duodenum is the initial part of the small intestine. The upper end connects to the pylorus of the stomach and the lower connects with jejunum at the duodenojejunal flexure. The duodenum bends like "C" shaped, wrapped around the head of the pancreas. It is divided into four parts: the upper part, the descending part, the horizontal part and the ascending part.

V. Answer the questions in detail

1. The extrahepatic bile duct is composed of the left and right hepatic ducts, common hepatic duct, common bile duct and gallbladder.

The gallbladder is located in the gallbladder fossa on inferior surface of the liver. It can be divided into four parts: the fundus, the body, the neck and the cystic duct. The fundus projects to the point of abdominal wall where the lateral border of right rectus abdominis (or right midclavicular line) crosses to the right costal arch.

The common hepatic duct is formed by the union of the right and left hepatic ducts. Then the common hepatic duct joins with the cystic duct to form the common bile duct. The common bile duct can be divided into four parts: the supraduodenal part (first segment), the retroduodenal part (second segment), the pancreatic part (third part) and the intraduodenal part (fourth part).

The thickened the circular muscles around the lower part of the common bile duct and the terminal part of pancreatic duct is called the sphincter of hepatopancreatic ampulla (or the sphincter of Oddi).

2. The stomach is in the epigastric and left hypochondriac regions of the abdomen. The cardiac orifice is on the left of the T_{11} vertebra. The pyloric orifice is just to the right of midline in a plane that passes through the lower border of vertebra L_1 (the transpyloric plane).

The anterior wall of the stomach on the right side is related to the left lobe of liver, left upper portion to the diaphragm and the lower portion to the anterior abdominal wall. The posterior wall of stomach contacts with the stomach bed (the diaphragm, left suprarenal gland, left kidney, pancreas, spleen, transverse colon and its mesocolon) by omental bursa.

The arterial supply to the stomach includes: the left gastric artery from the celiac trunk, the right gastric artery from the hepatic artery proper, the right gastroepiploic artery from the gastroduodenal artery, the left gastroepiploic artery from the splenic artery and the posterior gastric artery from the splenic artery (variant and not alwayspresent). The veins accompany with the same name arteries, drain into the hepatic portal vein finally.

There are left and right gastric lymph nodes, left and right gastroepiploic lymph nodes, cardiac nodes, superior and inferior pyloric lymph nodes, splenic lymph nodes. All of the efferent lymphatic ducts drain into the celiac lymph node.

The nerves to the stomach have the motor fibers and sensory fibers. The sympathetic never comes from the $T_6 \sim T_{10}$, and the parasympathetic nerve comes from the vagus nerve. The sensory fibers run within the sympathetic and parasympathetic nerves to the spinal cord or medulla.

Section 5   The Infracolic Compartment

Ⅰ. Single choice

1. A   2. D   3. B   4. A   5. B   6. B   7. D   8. C   9. C   10. A   11. B   12. D   13. D
14. C   15. D   16. B   17. A   18. B   19. C   20. D

Ⅱ. Double choices

1. DE   2. AE   3. DE   4. BC   5. BD   6. AC   7. DE   8. BC   9. CE   10. CE

Ⅲ. Fill the blanks

1. left of the L_2 vertebra; right sacroiliac joint; superior mesenteric

2. intestinal

3. left iliac crest, S_3 vertebra

4. ileocolic, superior mesenteric

5. ileocolic artery

6. McBurney's, Lanz

7. right colic flexure (hepatic flexure), left colic flexure (splenic flexure)

8. colic bands, haustra of colon, epiploic appendices

Ⅳ. Answer the questions briefly

1. The arteries of the colon include the ileocolic artery, right colic artery, middle colic artery, left colic artery and sigmoid arteries. The left colic artery and sigmoid arteries arise from the inferior mesenteric artery. The others arise from the superior mesenteric artery.

2. The hepatic portal vein is formed by the union of splenic vein and superior mesenteric vein behind the neck of pancreas. Then it passes upwards to the hilum of liver behind the superior part of duodenum and inside of the hepatoduodenal ligament. In addition, the other tributaries are the inferior mesenteric vein, left gastric vein, right gastric vein, paraumbilical vein and cystic vein.

3. The lymph of the jejunum and ileum is drained by lymphatic vessels along the blood vessels. Their lymph first passes through the mesenteric lymph nodes placed along the branches of the superior mesenteric artery, and then they converge to the superior mesenteric lymph nodes. Lastly, their efferent vessels enter into the intestinal lymphatic trunk.

4. The jejunum and ileum are supplied by autonomic nerves. The sympathetic fibers arise from celiac plexus, and the parasympathetic fivers arise from the vagus nerve. In superior mesenteric plexus, they send numerous branches accompanying the superior mesenteric artery and its branches to supply the jejunum and ileum.

5. The mesenteric triangle is located in the intestinal end of the mesentery and is bounded by the two layers peritoneum and the intestine wall at the mesenteric border. The intestine wall in this triangle is not covered by the peritoneum.

V. Answer the questions in detail

1. The vermiform appendix lies in the right inguinal region. The root of it is constant and its surface projection is McBurney's point or Lanz point. The McBurney's point lies at the junction of the middle and lateral thirds of a line from the umbilicus to the right anterior superior iliac spine. The Lanz point is a junction of the right and middle thirds of a line between both sides of anterior superior iliac spine.

The root of vermiform appendix is constant and it attaches to the posteromedial wall of the cecum, 2 – 3 cm below the ileocecal valve, where threes colic bands unite. According to this, the vermiform appendix can be found in abdominal cavity.

2. The jejunum occupies the upper 2/5 and locates in the upper left abdominal cavity near to the umbilical region. However, the ileum occupies lower 3/5 of small intestine and lies in the lower right abdominal cavity near to the hypogastric region.

The arteries of jejunum and ileum are the branches of the superior mesenteric artery. Before into the intestine, the branches of jejunum form 1 – 2 series of arterial arches while branches of ileum form 3 – 4 series of arterial arches.

The jejunum is thicker, redder and has more blood vessels than ileum. The circular folds of jejunum are larger in size, more in number than ileum. The jejunum only has solitary lymphatic follicles whereas the ileum has both solitary lymphatic follicles and aggregated lymphatic follicles.

3. There are three main collateral anastomoses between the hepatic portal vein and the systemic vein. Firstly, at the esophageal venous plexus, the left gastric vein of the hepatic portal system communicates with the esophageal vein, hemiazygos vein and azygos vein of superior vena cava system. Secondly, at the rectal venous plexus, the superior rectal vein of the hepatic portal system anastomoses with the inferior rectal vein and anal vein of the inferior vena cava system. Lastly, at the periumbilical venous plexus, the paraumbilical vein of the hepatic portal vein communicates with the thoracoepigastric vein and superior epigastric vein of the superior vena cava system. Meanwhile, paraumbilical vein anastomoses with the superficial epigastric vein and inferior epigastric vein of the inferior vena cava system through periumbilical venous rete.

In portal hypertension, some of the portal drainages may then back up and pass through the portal-systemic anastomoses in a reverse direction.

Section 6   The Retroperitoneal Space

I. Single choice

1. B   2. D   3. A   4. B   5. C   6. D   7. A   8. D   9. C   10. C

II. Double choices

1. CD   2. CE   3. BC   4. CD   5. AC

III. Fill the blanks

1. superior border of the T_{12}, superior border of the L_3

2. inferior border of the T_{11}, inferior border of the L_2

3. renal fascia, adipose capsule, fibrous capsule

4. renal vein, renal artery, renal pelvis

5. renal plexus, renal artery

6. inferior phrenic artery, abdominal aorta, renal artery

7. right common iliac vein, left common iliac vein, L_5

8. celiac trunk, superior mesenteric artery, inferior mesenteric artery

9. inferior vena cava, left renal vein

10. abdominal aorta, celiac trunk, superior mesenteric artery

IV. Answer the questions briefly

1. The retroperitoneal space is between the parietal peritoneum and endoabdominal fascia of posterior abdominal wall. Its superior boundary is diaphragm and inferior boundary is sacral promontory and pelvic inlet. The main structures in the space include kidney, ureter, adrenal gland, abdominal aorta, inferior vena cava, sympathetic trunk, etc.

2. The arteries of suprarenal gland include superior, middle and inferior suprarenal arteries. The superior one arises from the inferior phrenic artery. The middle one arises from abdominal aorta directly and the inferior one arises from the renal artery. There is one suprarenal vein in each side. The left suprarenal vein drains into the left renal vein whereas the right suprarenal vein drains into the inferior vena cava directly.

3. Anterior to the upper part of the right ureter are the descending part of duodenum, right colic and ileocolic arteries, root of the mesentery and right testicular (ovarian) vessels; in front of the lower part are the ileocecum and vermiform appendix. In front of the left one are duodenojejunal flexure, left colic artery, left testicular (ovarian) vessels and sigmoid mesocolon.

V. Answer the questions in detail

1. The abdominal aorta is the main vessel in the retroperitoneal space. It is continuous with the thoracic aorta at the level of 12th thoracic vertebra (the aortic hiatus of diaphragm), then it runs downward in front of the vertebral column, then bifurcates into right and left common iliac arteries at the lower border of L_4.

The parietal branches include inferior phrenic arteries, lumbar arteries and the median sacral artery.

The single visceral branches include the celiac trunk, superior mesenteric artery and the inferior mesenteric artery.

The paired visceral branches include the middle suprarenal artery, the renal artery and the testicular (ovarian) artery.

2. The kidneys are extra-peritoneal organs and located in the retroperitoneal space. They

lie in the paravertebral gutters. The right kidney is $1-2$ cm lower than the left because of the liver.

The right kidney: between superior borders of $T_{12}-L_3$ vertebrae, and the 12th rib passing through its upper part posteriorly.

The left kidney: between inferior borders of $T_{11}-L_2$ vertebrae, and the 12th rib passing through its middle part posteriorly.

The renal angle is on the posterior abdominal wall and is bounded by the lateral edge of erector spines and the 12th rib. The surface projection of renal hilum is on the anterior end of the 9th rib anteriorly and on renal angle posteriorly.

There aresuprarenal glands superiorly. There are diaphragm, 12th rib, subcostal nerve, iliohypogastric nerve, ilioinguinal nerve, genitofemoral nerve, psoas major and quadratus lumborum posterior to the kidneys. The structure medially to the left kidney is abdominal aorta, inferior vena cava to right kidney. Anteriorly there are stomach, pancreas, jejunum and left colic flexure to left kidney; right lobe of liver, right colic flexure and descending part of duodenum to right kidney.

The coverings of kidney include the renal fascia, adipose capsule and fibrous capsule form outside in. The adipose capsule is also named "renal bed".

Chapter 7　The Pelvis and Perineum

Section 1　Introduction

I . **Single choice**

    1. D 2. A 3. C

II . **Double choices**

    1. DE 2. AE

III . **Fill the blanks**

    1. anal region, urogenital region

    2. greater(false) pelvis, lesser(true) pelvis

IV . **Answer the questions briefly**

The perineum is the part of trunk below the pelvic diaphragm and has the same boundaries as the outlet of pelvis. The lateral boundaries are the inferior rami of the pubes, the rami of ischia and the sacrotuberous ligaments. A line joining the ischial tuberosities divides the perineum into posterior anal region and anterior urogenital region.

Section 2   The Pelvis

Ⅰ. Single choice

1. A   2. B   3. C   4. B   5. C   6. D   7. A   8. D   9. D   10. B   11. A   12. A   13. D
14. B   15. B   16. B   17. D   18. B   19. C   20. C   21. C   22. C   23. C   24. D   25. D   26. D

Ⅱ. Double choices

1. AE   2. CD   3. BE   4. AB   5. BC   6. CD   7. CE   8. BC   9. AD   10. CE   11. CD

Ⅲ. Fill the blanks

1. obturator internus, piriformis

2. sacrotuberous ligament, sacrospinous ligament

3. obturator canal

4. 4th lumbar vertebra; external iliac artery, internal iliac artery

5. deep iliac circumflex artery, inferior epigastric artery

6. obturator artery, inferior gluteal artery

7. ganglion impar, four

8. ureteric orifices, internal urethral orifice

9. internal pudendal artery, dentate line

10. inferior mesenteric lymph nodes, internal iliac lymph nodes, superficial inguinal lymph nodes

11. Sympathetic, parasympathetic, anale

12. anteflexion

13. supravaginal, vaginal

14. uterine part, isthmus, ampulla, infundibulum

15. mesovarium

Ⅳ. Answer the questions briefly

1. The uterine tube lies in the upper border of the broad ligament. Each connects the peritoneal cavity with the cavity of the uterus. It is divided into four parts. From medial-laterally, they are the uterine part, isthmus, ampulla and infundibulum. The ampulla is the widest part of the tube where fertilization of the ovum can take place. The isthmus is the narrowest part of the tube where the ligation of the uterine tube is performed usually.

2. The lymph vessels of the rectum drain first into the pararectal lymph nodes and then into inferior mesenteric lymph nodes. Lymph vessels from the lower part of the rectum follow the inferior rectal artery to the internal iliac lymph nodes.

3. The pelvic fascia can be divided into parietal pelvic fascia, viscera pelvic fascia and fascia of the pelvic diaphragm.

Parietal fascia covers the anterior, posterior and lateral walls of the pelvis as well as the obturator internus and piriformis. The visceral pelvic fascia covers the organs, blood vessels, and nerves in the pelvis. Some fascial coverings form capsules around organs; in some places, the fascia is thickened to form ligaments. Between some organs, the visceral fascia forms fascial septum. The fascia of pelvic diaphragm lines the floor of the pelvis named the superior and inferior fascia of pelvic diaphragm.

4. The urinary bladder is situated in the pelvis behind the pubis. Its shape and relations vary according to the amount of urine that it contains. The empty bladder in the adult lies entirely within the pelvis; as the bladder fills, its superior wall rises up into the hypogastric region.

The empty bladder is pyramidal, having an apex, a fundus, a neck and a body. The apex of the bladder points anteriorly and lies behind the upper margin of the symphysis pubis. The fundus faces posteriorly and is triangular. The body is the part between the apex and fundus. The lowest and most fixed part is the neck of bladder. It has 4 surfaces: superior, two inferolateral and posterior(fundus) surfaces.

5. The anterior trunk of internal iliac artery has two kinds of branches, the parietal and visceral branches. The parietal branches are the obturator artery and inferior gluteal artery. The visceral branches are the umbilical artery, inferior vesical artery, inferior rectal artery, internal pudendal artery and uterine artery.

6. The ovary usually lies against the lateral wall of the pelvis in a depression called the ovarian fossa, bounded by the external iliac vessels above and the internal iliac vessels behind. The ovarian artery arises from the abdominal aorta at the level of the 1st lumbar vertebra. The ovarian vein drains into the inferior vena cava on the right side and into the left renal vein on the left side.

V. Answer the questions in detail

1. **Location**: The rectum begins in front of the third sacral vertebra as a continuation of the sigmoid colon. It passes downward, following the curve of the sacrum and coccyx, and ends in front of the tip of the coccyx by piercing the pelvic diaphragm and becoming continuous with the anal canal.

Relations: Posteriorly: The rectum is in contact with the sacrum and coccyx; the piriformis, coccygeus, and levatores ani muscles; the sacral plexus; the sympathetic trunks. Anteriorly: In the male, the upper two thirds of the rectum, which is covered by peritoneum, is related to the sigmoid colon and coils of ileum that occupy the rectovesical pouch. The lower third of the rectum is related to the posterior surface of the bladder, the termination of the ductus deferens and the seminal vesicles on each side, and to the prostate. In the female, the upper two thirds of the rectum is related to the sigmoid colon and coils of ileum that occupy the rectouterine pouch (pouch of Douglas). The lower third of the rectum is related to the posterior surface of the vagina.

Blood supply: Arteries: The superior and inferior rectal arteries and anal artery supply the rectum. The superior rectal artery is a direct continuation of the inferior mesenteric artery. It divides into right and left branches, entering the lateral wall of the tectum. The inferior rectal artery is a branch of the internal iliac artery supplying the lower part of the rectum. The anal artery is a branch of the internal pudendal artery supplying the part of anal canal below the dentate line. Veins: The accompanying veins begin from the venous plexus of the rectum. The internal rectal venous plexus drains into the superior rectal vein which drains into the portal system, via the inferior mesenteric vein. The external rectal venous plexus drains into the inferior rectal vein and anal vein, then into the internal iliac vein.

2. **Location**: In normal condition, the uterus extends between the bladder and the rectum in the pelvic cavity. The long axis of the uterus is bent forward on the long axis of the vagina. This position is referred to as anteversion of the uterus. The long axis of the body of the uterus is bent forward with the long axis of the cervix. This position is termed anteflexion of the uterus.

Relation: Anteriorly: The body of the uterus is related anteriorly to the uterovesical pouch and the superior surface of the bladder. The supravaginal part of cervix is related to the superior surface of the bladder. The vaginal part of cervix is related to the anterior fornix of the vagina. Posteriorly: The body of the uterus is related posteriorly to the rectouterine pouch (pouch of Douglas) with coils of ileum or sigmoid colon within it. Laterally: The body of the uterus is related laterally to the broad ligament and the uterine artery and vein. The supravaginal part of cervix is related to the ureter as it passes forward to enter the bladder. The vaginal part of cervix is related to the lateral fornix of the vagina. The uterine tubes enter the superolateral angles of the uterus, and the round ligaments of the ovary and of the uterus are attached to the uterine wall just below this level.

Supports structures: The uterus is supported mainly by the major muscles of the pelvic floor, neighboring organs and connective tissues and several ligaments: ① Broad ligament of uterus: It is situated in coronal plane and stretches from the lateral margin of the uterus to the side wall of pelvis. ②Round ligament of uterus: It extends between the superolateral angle of the uterus, through the deep inguinal ring and inguinal canal, to the subcutaneous tissue of the labium majus. It helps to keep the uterus anteverted and anteflexed. ③Cardinal ligament of uterus: It is composed of connective tissue passing laterally from side of the neck to the side wall of pelvis. It maintains the uterus in its normal position and prevents the prolapse. ④Uterosacral ligament: It consists of two firm fibromuscular bands of pelvic fascia that pass to the cervix from the lower end of the sacrum.

Section 3　The Perineum

Ⅰ. Single choice

1. B　2. B　3. D　4. C　5. D　6. B　7. D　8. B　9. A　10. C　11. A　12. C　13. B
14. D　15. D　16. C　17. D　18. C　19. B　20. D　21. A　22. C　23. C　24. B　25. C

II . Double choices

1. BD   2. AB   3. BD   4. DE   5. BE   6. DE   7. BC   8. BD   9. DE   10. AB

III . Fill the blanks

1. fatty, membranous

2. subcutaneous part, superficial part, deep part

3. superior fascia of urogenital diaphragm, inferior fascia of urogenital diaphragm, deep transverse muscle of perineum

IV . Answer the questions briefly

1. The urogenital diaphragm lies in the anterior part of the perineum. It is formed by the sphincter urethra, and deep transverse perineal muscles, which are enclosed by superior and inferior fasciae of urogenital diaphragm.

2. In male, it contains membranous part of urethra, sphincter urethrae, bulbourethral glands, deep transverse perineal muscle, internal pudendal vessels and their branches, and dorsal nerves of the penis. In female, it contains part of urethra, part of vagina, sphincter urethra, deep transverse perineal muscle, internal pudendal vessels and their branches, dorsal nerves of clitoris.

3. The wall of scrotum contains skin, dartos coat, external spermatic fascia, cremaster, internal spermatic fascia and tunica vaginalis of testis.

4. The anal canal has 2 kinds of sphincters, involuntary internal sphincter, and voluntary external sphincter. The sphincter ani internus is the thickened linner circular smooth muscle around the upper two-thirds of the anal canal. The sphincter ani externus has three parts which are distinctly separated from each other. The subcutaneous part surrounds the anus. It has no bony attachment, but its fibers decussate anteriorly to the perineal central tendon and posteriorly the anococcygeal ligament. The superficial part is oval in shape, its fibers arise from the coccyx and pass anteriorly around the anus to the perineal central tendon. The deep part is fused with the puborectal part of the levator ani which reinforces its action.

5. The spermatic cord suspends the testis in the scrotum and extends from the deep inguinal ring to the posterior aspect of the testis. In the inguinal canal, the spermatic cord acquires coverings from the layers of the abdominal wall that extend into the scrotal wall as the internal spermatic fascia, cremaster, and external spermatic fascia. The internal spermatic fascia is derived from the transverse fascia. The cremaster is continuous with obliquus internus abdominis and transversus abdominis. The external spermatic fascia descends from the aponeurosis of obliquus externus abdominis. The spermatic cord contains the ductus deferens, testicular artery, pampiniform plexus of vein, genital branch of the genitofemoral nerve, lymphatic vessels and the remnants of the vaginal process.

V . Answer the questions in detail

1. **Formation:** It is the space between the Colles' fascia and the inferior fascia of urogeni-

tal diaphragm. It is closed behind by the fusion of its upper and lower walls. Laterally, it is closed by the attachment of its upper and lower walls to the pubic arch.

Contents: In female, there are superficial transverse muscles of perineum, bulbocavernosus, ischiocavernosus, bulb of vestibule, crus of clitoris, greater vestibular glands, nerves and blood vessels to supply the perineum. In male, there are superficial transverse muscles of perineum, bulbocavernosus, ischiocavernosus, bulb of urethra, crus of penis, nerves and blood vessels to supply the perineum.

2. **Location:** The ischioanal fossa is a wedge-shaped space located on each side of the anal canal.

Boundaries: Its apex lies superiorly, and the base is the perineal skin. The medial wall is formed by the levator ani, sphincter ani externus and the inferior fascia of pelvic diaphragm. The lateral wall is formed by the ischial tuberosity, sacrotuberous ligament and the fascia of obturator internus. Posteriorly the fossa is bounded by the gluteus maximus and the sacrotuberous ligament. This fossa extends forwards above the urogenital diaphragm and backwards deep to the gluteus maximus.

Contents: It contains fat, branches of pudendal nerve and internal pudendal vessels.

3. The male urethra extends from the neck of the bladder to the external meatus on the glans penis. It is divided into three parts: prostatic, membranous and cavernous.

The prostaticpart of urethra passes through the prostate from the base to the apex. It is the widest and most dilatable portion of the urethra. On its posterior wall, there are the urethral crest, prostatic sinus, seminal colliculus and the openings of ejaculatory ducts.

The membranous part of urethra lies within the urogenital diaphragm, surrounded by the sphincter urethra. It is the least dilatable portion of the urethra.

The cavernous part of urethra is enclosed in the bulb and the cavernous body of the penis. The external orifice is the narrowest part of the entire urethra. The part of the urethra that lies within the glans penis is dilated to form the navicular fossa. The bulbourethral glands open into the cavernous part of urethra below the urogenital diaphragm.

Chapter 8   The Back and Vertebral Region

Section 1   Introduction

I. Single choice

1. C   2. C

II. Answer the questions briefly

Its superior boundary is external occipital protuberance and superior nuchal line and inferior border is the line from the coccyx apex to posterior superior iliac spine. Its lateral border is anterior border of trapezius, posterior border of deltoid and posterior axillary line. It can be divided into the nape, the back, the lumbar and sacrococcygeal regions.

Section 2   The Layers and Structures

Ⅰ. Single choice

    1. A   2. D   3. D   4. D.   5. C   6. C

Ⅱ. Double choices

    1. AB   2. AE

Section 3   The Vertebral Canal and Its Contents

Ⅰ. Single choice

    1. B   2. D   3. D   4. C

Ⅱ. Answer the questions briefly

It is the interval between the arachnoid and pia mater, it contains the CSF and is traversed by connective tissue trabeculae. The space becomes wider from the lower end of spinal cord to the second sacral vertebra, which is called terminal cistern and contains the cauda equina. Terminal cistern is the best site for a lumbar puncture because of avoiding injury to the spinal cord.

References

[1] WANG HUAIJING. Regional Anatomy[M]. 5th edition. Changchun: Jilin Science and Technology Press, 2009.

[2] KEITH L MOOR, ARTHUR F DALLEY, ANNE M R AGUR. Clinically Oriente Anatomy[M]. 6th Edition. Philadelphia: Lippincott Williams & Wilkins, 2010.

[3] RICHARD L DRAKE, A WAYNE VOGL, ADAM W M MITCHELL. Gray's Basic Anatomy[M]. Peking: Peking University Medical Press, 2013.